CHAIN ANALYSIS ...CAL
BEHAVIOR ...

Guilford DBT® Practice Series
Alan E. Fruzzetti, *Series Editor*

This series presents accessible, step-by-step guides to essential components of dialectical behavior therapy (DBT) practice. Delving deeply into different aspects of DBT implementation—phone coaching, validation, chain analysis, family interventions, and more—series volumes distill the latest clinical innovations and provide practical help based on sound DBT principles and good science.

Phone Coaching in Dialectical Behavior Therapy
Alexander L. Chapman

Chain Analysis in Dialectical Behavior Therapy
Shireen L. Rizvi

DBT® Teams: Development and Practice
Jennifer H. R. Sayrs and Marsha M. Linehan

Chain Analysis in Dialectical Behavior Therapy

Shireen L. Rizvi

Series Editor's Note by Alan E. Fruzzetti

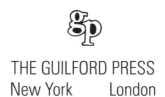

THE GUILFORD PRESS
New York   London

Library of Congress Cataloging-in-Publication Data

Names: Rizvi, Shireen L., author.
Title: Chain analysis in dialectical behavior therapy / Shireen L. Rizvi.
Other titles: Guilford DBT practice series.
Description: New York : The Guilford Press, 2019. | Series: Guilford DBT
    practice series | Includes bibliographical references and index.
Identifiers: LCCN 2018053815 | ISBN 9781462538904 (paperback) |
    ISBN 9781462538911 (hardcover)
Subjects: | MESH: Behavior Therapy—methods
Classification: LCC RC489.B4 | NLM WM 425 | DDC 616.89/142—dc23
LC record available at https://lccn.loc.gov/2018053815

DBT is a registered trademark of Marsha M. Linehan. Marsha M. Linehan has
not participated in the preparation of this book.

About the Author

Shireen L. Rizvi, PhD, ABPP, is Associate Professor of Clinical Psychology in the Graduate School of Applied and Professional Psychology at Rutgers, The State University of New Jersey. At Rutgers, she holds affiliate appointments in the Department of Psychology, School of Arts and Sciences, and the Department of Psychiatry, Robert Wood Johnson Medical School. Her research interests include improving outcomes, training, and dissemination of dialectical behavior therapy (DBT) for the treatment of complex and severe problems. Dr. Rizvi is board certified in Behavioral and Cognitive Psychology and in Dialectical Behavior Therapy. She is past president of the International Society for the Improvement and Teaching of DBT and was the Society's Conference Program Chair for 2 years. She has trained hundreds of practitioners from around the world in DBT. Dr. Rizvi is a recipient of the Spotlight on a Mentor Award from the Association of Behavioral and Cognitive Therapies and the Presidential Fellowship for Teaching Excellence from Rutgers.

Series Editor's Note

DIALECTICAL BEHAVIOR THERAPY—THEN AND NOW

This excellent book on chain analysis is the second book in the Guilford DBT® Practice Series, which was developed to meet the increasing needs of practitioners to learn how to do dialectical behavior therapy (DBT) well—in an adherent and competent way. DBT was developed originally for suicidal and/or self-harming patients with borderline personality and related disorders. While the DBT treatment manual (Linehan, 1993a), the revised *DBT Skills Training Manual* (Linehan, 2015b), and the *DBT Skills Training Handouts and Worksheets* (Linehan 2015a) provide therapists with the entire treatment protocol, other aspects of the treatment—chain analysis, validation, phone coaching, family interventions, consultation team, and effective use of dialectical strategies, to name a few—have developed considerably beyond the original treatment manual. It is for this reason that we developed this series, with the support of Dr. Marsha M. Linehan, to help practitioners enhance and refine their skills and deliver DBT to their patients more effectively, according to present DBT standards and practices.

When the young psychologist Marsha Linehan and her colleagues at the University of Washington developed DBT in the 1980s, it was not at all clear if the treatment would be successful, in terms of both treatment efficacy for people who are chronically suicidal and self-harming (typically referred to as having borderline personality disorder, or BPD), for whom the treatment was developed, and acceptance and adoption for use by the therapeutic community, who long had struggled to treat people with these problems. In order to understand how the accessible guides in this series enhance the literature and promote adherence to current DBT principles and practices, we must first show how they fit into the overall structure of DBT treatment and the treatment context for BPD and related problems that has evolved over time.

Looking back 30 years or more, it is stunning to see the impact Dr. Linehan's work has had on the field. Before her work became widely disseminated and accepted, suicidal and/or self-harming people with BPD faced rampant stigmatization, a sense of hopelessness about recovery, and a complete absence of empirically supported treatments. Needless to say, people with BPD faced a bleak prognosis. At the time, DBT was available only in a small clinic at the University of Washington. There was no treatment manual or skills manual; there were no clear ways to teach, disseminate, or implement the treatment effectively.

Where are we now? Stigma has been significantly reduced, hope has increased, there is a general recognition among professionals that BPD and related problems are treatable (although there is still a long way to go), and an impressive volume of studies demonstrate strong support for BPD's efficacy and effectiveness. There is a widely read treatment manual (Linehan, 1993a), and both an original (1993b) and enhanced and updated skills manual (2015a, 2015b). Well-trained teams in outpatient, residential, hospital, and other settings treat thousands of people every day with DBT, not only across the United States but in dozens of countries and on every continent. Many of these treatment providers have demonstrated both their commitment and their abilities by becoming certified as DBT therapists, which requires rigorous demonstration of their skills as DBT providers. In addition, other effective treatments, generally also nonpejorative toward people with BPD and related difficulties, have been empirically established or are under development.

Moreover, applications and adaptations of DBT have been successfully developed for a host of problems other than BPD per se (i.e., other severe problems related to emotion dysregulation) and across a variety of treatment—and, more recently, prevention—settings. It's not a surprise that Dr. Linehan was recently featured as one of the 100 "Great Scientists" of all time ("Great Scientists," 2018).

DBT is an *integrative* treatment that includes a whole set of interventions (modes and functions of treatment). DBT includes not only individual therapy but also multiple other modalities that serve different functions in treatment, such as group skills training, telephone coaching, family interventions, and an ongoing consultation team. DBT integrates the techniques and scope of acceptance-oriented therapies (e.g., support, warmth, encouragement) with the strategies and precision of behavior therapies and emotion science (e.g., precise treatment targets, scientific analysis of behavior [emotions, thoughts, actions]) and focuses on psychological and social skills as *solutions* to a range of problems. Dozens of controlled studies support the effectiveness of DBT in creating safety, stability, and self-control while minimizing treatment dropout, as well as improving mood, self-esteem, relationships, family, school and job functioning, and so forth. Largely due to stable outcomes and reduced relapse, costs of DBT compared to alternative treatments are also significantly reduced in the long term.

The DBT Model

The treatment model views *emotion dysregulation* as the core of a variety of emotional, cognitive (thinking), relational, identity (self-concept), and behavioral problems. Emotion dysregulation increases or exacerbates behavioral dysregulation (out-of-control actions, including impulsivity), cognitive dysregulation (trouble thinking and problem solving), interpersonal dysregulation (difficulties in relationships), and self-dysregulation (problems with self-esteem, identity, negative self-views). Consequently, many common co-occurring problems (suicidal and nonsuicidal self-injury, depression, anxiety, eating disorders, posttraumatic stress disorder, substance abuse, aggression, problems in relationships, etc.) are similarly understood either as dysfunctional attempts to regulate emotion or as natural consequences of chronic emotion dysregulation. The overarching goal of DBT is to help people create lives worth living by helping them learn psychological and social skills to regulate, or manage, their emotions—earlier in treatment tolerating and re-regulating secondary emotions, and later in treatment identifying, accurately labeling, allowing, expressing accurately, and managing primary emotions. Much of the treatment is built around these principles.

Chronic and severe emotion dysregulation is hypothesized to result from an ongoing *transaction* between the person's emotion vulnerabilities and ongoing invalidation from others in the social and family environment, which often promotes self-invalidation as well. Emotion vulnerability is influenced by temperament, conditioning, and present biological disposition resulting from learning and current circumstances and manifests as emotional sensitivity and reactivity, along with often slow return to emotion equilibrium. Invalidating responses can take a variety of forms, from the obviously critical and emotionally abusive to well-meaning misunderstandings that occur because of temperamental differences, inaccurate expression, or miscommunication between people and their family members and others.

Five Core Functions of Comprehensive DBT

DBT consists of components or modes that address the five essential functions of treatment:

1. Help people learn new psychological, emotional, and social/ relationship skills, typically via skills training groups.

2. Help people generalize those skills to their real, everyday lives, in situations that have elicited less skillful responses in the past, which includes detailed planning, *in vivo* coaching, and practicing skills in the "real" world.

3. Help people collaborate on their treatment targets and enhance their motivation to replace overlearned dysfunctional behaviors with more skillful alternatives, primarily through individual psychotherapy, and also in other ways, depending on treatment setting.

4. Help people manage their social and family relationships to build better relationships and elicit more support, understanding, and validation and help family members become more validating and supportive in return.

5. Provide ongoing support, validation, problem solving, and skill building for therapists to enhance their motivation and skills through regular team consultation meetings.

DBT Skills

Learning key psychological, emotional, and social skills is believed to be central in helping patients learn to regulate their emotions, build satisfying relationships, and thrive. These include skills to:

1. Increase attention control and nonjudgmental awareness and build a more positive self-concept or identity (mindfulness).

2. Understand emotions, increase positive emotions, decrease vulnerability to negative reactions, accept negative emotional experiences, and change negative emotional experiences (emotion regulation skills).

3. Build empathy and improve relationships while balancing assertion with self-respect (interpersonal skills).

4. Tolerate highly distressing experiences without doing things impulsively that increase dysregulation overall (distress tolerance skills).

5. Balance competing goals, interests, and perspectives and build cognitive and emotional flexibility (dialectics, or the middle path, along with "wise mind").

Over time, some additional skills have become part of the DBT lexicon, such as dialectical and validation skills for patients and their families, specific skills for people with substance use problems, and so on (cf. Fruzzetti, Payne, & Hoffman, in press; Miller, Rathus, & Linehan, 2007; Rathus & Miller, 2015).

Of course, principles of learning are at the core of any behavior therapy, including DBT. In particular, there are three overlapping phases of learning: (1) the acquisition phase, in which the basics of the skill are learned, typically in skills training groups designed to be optimal learning environments; (2) the strengthening phase, in which the person practices the skill, typically in planned ways, in groups or with the therapist or at home; and (3) the generalization phase, in which the person's skill has become robust enough that he or she can employ it when needed in his or her life, often spontaneously. Of course, in addition to the teaching/training and coaching that occur in skills training groups and in individual sessions, in outpatient settings *in vivo* coaching can help to generalize skills (mostly by text or telephone) and manage between-session problems.

Acceptance and Validation

Throughout DBT, treatment providers strive to understand and validate the primary emotional experience of their patients, along with other valid behaviors, and help clients validate themselves. We do not validate things that are not, in fact, valid. This is a complex task, learning to discriminate the valid aspects of any given behavior from the invalid ones. For example, certain impulsive and/or destructive behaviors (e.g., self-harm, substance use) are typically primary targets for change because they are invalid ways to solve problems or enhance quality of life in the long term. Yet, they are valid in the sense that they do often "work" to reduce, avoid, or escape painful negative emotional arousal, albeit briefly. Understanding and validating what is valid, even in the most dysfunctional behavior, is a key therapeutic activity that helps the client feel understood (validated), increases motivation for change, builds the therapeutic relationship, and thus increases collaboration for change. Consequently, therapist validation not only has value in itself (feeling understood, cared about, etc.), it also helps regulate the person and promotes change.

Change, Problem Solving, and Behavior Therapy

Within a therapeutic context based on understanding, acceptance, and validation, the therapist targets dysfunctional behaviors for change, pushing patients to substitute skillful alternatives for the problematic reactions and dysfunctional behaviors for which they sought treatment. Utilizing a carefully constructed treatment target hierarchy, DBT therapists and the DBT team can employ all the components of learning and behavior therapy: (1) careful assessment, using chain analysis; (2) development of solutions on the chain and replacement of dysfunctional "links" in the chain that led to a dysfunctional or undesired behavior with a skillful alternative (this includes learning skills, noted above); (3) behavioral rehearsal and other commitment strategies to foster the difficult change process; and (4) all the techniques of behavior therapy to help the person actually use the skill when needed (e.g., stimulus control, reinforcement/contingency management, exposure and response prevention).

Dialectics

Balancing acceptance and validation with change, problem solving, and behavior therapy is complicated, and there are no algorithms to guide us because each context is unique. Rather, the therapist must balance these dialectically in the service of effectiveness. Every strategy in DBT has an "opposite" of equal value that must be considered and balanced in order to help people change in the ways they want to change. Just as acceptance and validation must be balanced with change and problem solving, intervening on behalf of clients is balanced by consulting with clients to empower them to intervene on their own behalf; communicating in a warm, genuine, and caring way must be balanced with irreverence, insistence, and matter-of-fact communication; and emotion must be balanced with reason (and vice versa).

Interventions in the Social and Family Environments

Although an important component of DBT from the beginning, social and family interventions are areas that have shown enormous growth and development since the first wave of DBT was developed and implemented. For example, fully developed applications of DBT have been shown to be effective with parents, couples, and families, and in school systems, and are being used to prevent the development of emotion dysregulation problems or to intervene early to help clients avoid full-blown problems related to emotion dysregulation. All of these efforts utilize the core principles of DBT, but of course have expanded the strategies and techniques to be effective in these new domains. Their growth and development are a positive testament to the coherence and effectiveness of DBT from the beginning.

What DBT Is and What It Is Not

Given the strong empirical foundation for DBT, it is no surprise that many clinicians want to offer DBT as part of their therapeutic toolbox. However, DBT is complex and requires considerable time, effort, and dedication to learn well. So, it is also not surprising that a wide range of treatments are offered under the DBT "label," but are of varying DBT quality. This is confusing for consumers at best, and of course fraudulent at worst. Imagine if a surgeon thought, "I've never had the training to do this procedure, but I read a little bit about it, so I can advertise myself as an expert in it." No one would want this surgeon performing a procedure on them. Fortunately, a certification process for DBT therapists, and their DBT teams, is now underway. This is a significant positive development both for people who need treatment (they will know what they are getting) and for DBT therapists (they will have objective measures that show they are doing excellent work).

How This Book Series Fits into the Development of DBT

DBT is, at least metaphorically, a living, breathing, and always growing and evolving treatment. It expands and changes in a dialectical manner. We use the therapy according to the model (the "thesis" or "proposition"); when something is not working well, DBT therapists innovate within the treatment ("antithesis" in which we employ theory and science to develop something new). In response to data and research findings about these innovations, we find some things work and others do not; ultimately, some new strategies or interventions become established and integrated with the old (synthesis, now established treatment), and stay that way until a situation arises in which they do not work well, and then further innovation (further antitheses) is engaged.

The original text (Linehan, 1993a) remains relevant and wise and includes an enormous amount of thoughtful and effective guidance. DBT has evolved since 1993 to include many more things (applications in new settings, extensions of principles and strategies, new skills, etc.) that could not have been anticipated at the time the book was written. This book series presents DBT as it is today, synthesizing the old and the new, built on the original treatment manual.

For example, the first book in this series (Chapman, 2019) focuses on telephone consultation with clients. This idea of coaching suicidal and self-harming clients by telephone between sessions was an innovative notion and was greeted by many therapists as a potentially frightening aspect of treatment. Were clients going to abuse their phone privileges, intrude on therapists' lives, and make never-ending demands on therapists' time? This book shows how to observe therapeutic limits, coach but not provide treatment, and use phone time to effectively advance treatment. We have learned a great deal about the nuances of skill coaching on the telephone, how the call might be different for teens than they are for adults, and other aspects of phone coaching that only emerged over time with much effort, innovation, and empirical evaluation.

Shireen Rizvi's book, the second book in the series, focuses on chain analysis and, by extension, solution analysis. Dr. Rizvi is truly an expert in DBT overall, and in chain and solution analysis in particular. A former doctoral student of Marsha Linehan at the University of Washington, she is now Associate Professor at Rutgers University, where she teaches, runs a DBT outpatient clinic, supervises novice DBT therapists, and conducts important research on various aspects of DBT. Given her enormous expertise, it is not surprising that this volume contains helpful information, specific instructions, tips, and a good deal of wisdom born of experience about chain analysis and solution analysis from beginning to end. In addition, this book provides myriad examples, transcripts of chain analyses, and essential guidance for effective practice.

Chain analyses provide the structure of DBT. That is, once we know what the problems (or primary targets) of the client are, doing a chain analysis is the way we begin to understand both the client's experience and the variables that control, or influence, the primary targets. DBT is a treatment grounded in mindfulness, and chain analysis requires careful observation and description of the factors that likely led to a particular episode of a primary target. Notice that we do not say the chain "caused" the behavior, because prior learning is understood to provide the largest share of causality. Thus, chains require careful, unbiased attention, observation, and description, and thus also provide mindfulness practice in self-awareness for the client. So, in these ways, chain analysis starts out as an "acceptance" intervention: The therapist and client endeavor simply to understand the problem behavior.

Of course, one of the key purposes of understanding the steps, or the chain of events and behaviors (including thoughts and emotions) that led to the problem behavior, is to help the client weave nascent skills into this and, more importantly, future chains. By identifying skills as solutions and practicing them, clients develop awareness, self-control, and choices and become empowered to manage their emotions, interpersonal relationships, and a wide range of challenging situations in a skillful and effective manner. And as clients become more mindful and aware of their thoughts, judgments, emotional reactions, urges, and so on, they discover more ways to access and use an ever-wider range of skills. In these ways, chain analysis and solution analysis are key components of change and problem solving in DBT.

As the client and therapist figure out the chain collaboratively, the therapist is afforded the opportunity to understand both the client's experience in depth and the factors or variables that "control" the problem behavior, both antecedents and consequences. The client's experience typically includes emotional reactions and thoughts or judgments that, without patiently conducting a detailed chain analysis, might be deeply misunderstood and invalidated (and almost certainly have been invalidated in the past). In addition, by developing the ability to use their curiosity, observing, and describing skills while doing a chain, clients discover deeper understanding and express themselves more accurately, which provides the context for the therapist to understand and validate clients genuinely, at different levels of validation. Once again, chain analysis is a key springboard for acceptance and validation, even when the target might also include changing a problematic or dysfunctional behavior.

In DBT, the combination or synthesis of acceptance and validation with change and problem solving are considered the "primary dialectic." We pay a lot of attention to balancing acceptance and change, and chain and solution analyses provide the core elements that the therapist and client can use to find an effective synthesis that empowers the client and helps resolve often long-standing difficulties. Consequently, chain analysis might help the client and the therapist understand particularly problematic thoughts or judgments, emotional reactions, urges, or even behaviors that were "missing" on the chain.

Dr. Rizvi explains clearly how to do these kinds of chain analyses. She also walks through how chain and solution analyses evolve over time in treatment (e.g., as clients and therapists begin to understand and anticipate patterns), and how to become more efficient in doing chains as treatment progresses. These sections, like the rest of the volume, include many practical tips and rich clinical material, including detailed transcripts.

The methods for doing chain and solution analyses across modes of DBT are beautifully and thoroughly explained in ways that are relevant to a variety of situations because chains are not found only in work with clients individually (individual session, coaching situations, etc.). In fact, chain and solution analyses are important assessment tools and strategies (acceptance and change) on DBT consultation teams and other modes of DBT (e.g., group skills training, family interventions) wherever and whenever we want to understand a problem, and/or ultimately decrease a problem behavior or increase a behavior whose absence is a problem.

This book continues the tradition in the series of providing in-depth yet practical help in using a core element of DBT in ways that adhere to DBT principles and practices. It is essential reading for both novice DBT therapists and well-established DBT therapists precisely because it employs the principles of DBT throughout while providing practical instructions and examples. Moreover, this book will be invaluable to therapists who practice cognitive-behavioral therapy or other modalities who are interested in a more descriptive, less interpretive, kind of assessment approach. And, of course, the material in this book is entirely consistent with core DBT competencies, adherence in DBT (necessary for certification as a DBT therapist), and Linehan's initial treatment manual (1993a). Like this book, the entire series intends to augment, rather than replace, earlier core DBT manuals (Linehan, 1993a, 2015a, 2015b). Each book in the series will illustrate many new developments, guided by both clinical innovation and sound research, that constitute DBT today.

ALAN E. FRUZZETTI, PhD

References

Chapman, A. L. (2019). *Phone coaching in dialectical behavior therapy.* New York: Guilford Press.

Fruzzetti, A. E., Payne, L., & Hoffman, P. D. (in press). Dialectical behavior therapy with families. In L. A. Dimeff, K. Koerner, & S. Rizvi (Eds.), *Dialectical behavior therapy in clinical practice: Applications across disorders and settings* (2nd ed.). New York: Guilford Press.

Great scientists: The geniuses and visionaries who transformed our world. (2018). *Time (Special Edition).* New York: Time, Inc.

Linehan, M. M. (1993a). *Cognitive-behavioral treatment of borderline personality disorder.* New York: Guilford Press.

Linehan, M. M. (1993b). *Skills training manual for treating borderline personality disorder.* New York: Guilford Press.

Linehan, M. M. (2015a). *DBT skills training handouts and worksheets* (2nd ed.). New York: Guilford Press.

Linehan, M. M. (2015b). *DBT skills training manual* (2nd ed.). New York: Guilford Press.

Miller, A. L., & Rathus, J. H., & Linehan, M. M. (2007). *Dialectical behavior therapy with suicidal adolescents.* New York: Guilford Press.

Rathus, J. H., & Miller, A. L. (2015). *DBT skills manual for adolescents.* New York: Guilford Press.

Preface

first came to learn dialectical behavior therapy (DBT®) when I was
a research assistant at Stanford University in the mid-1990s. I was
hired to manage several multisite randomized controlled trials in the
field of eating disorders and had plans to apply to doctoral programs with
faculty who specialized in that field. About halfway through my time
there, I was asked to help coordinate a new pilot study conducted by Dr.
Christy Telch, an expert in eating disorders and specifically binge eating.
She had decided to examine an adaptation of DBT skills training for
individuals meeting criteria for binge-eating disorder. As a research assistant on this project, I became increasingly familiar with DBT through
reviewing skills worksheets and listening to audiotapes of the sessions.
I also became familiar with an assessment strategy known as the "chain
analysis," which Christy taught as a skill to her participants. I grew more
and more intrigued by this relatively new treatment, to the extent that I
began reading extensively about both the treatment and borderline personality disorder (BPD). My keen interest drove me to change directions
and apply to the clinical psychology PhD program at the University of
Washington in order to study with Marsha Linehan. Much to my delight,
I was accepted and proceeded to work with Marsha on a near-daily basis
for the subsequent 5 years.

   As my clinical supervisor for many years, Marsha met with me on a
weekly basis to discuss my DBT treatment cases and watch videos of my
sessions. A typical sequence in supervision would go like this: I would go
into her office, put in the VHS tape, press "play," about 5 seconds would

transpire, and Marsha would say, "Stop! [pause] Why did you say 'hello' like that?" Despite attempts to justify my tone and words, Marsha would find ways to show me how I could be more effective. She would model a response and then we would role-play so that I could get the experience of doing it "the Marsha way." We would turn on the video again, 10 seconds would transpire, and she would say, "Stop! Why did you do *that?*," and so on. I would later joke that I became an expert in how to do the first 5 minutes of a DBT therapy session. And although these first few minutes of a session are extremely important for setting the stage, it is what happens during the rest of the session that usually leads to the transformative changes in the individual's life. In fact, it is somewhat embarrassing for me to admit now, but it took nearly a year of intensive training in DBT for it to "click" about how all the complex pieces of DBT fit together to become a unified and effective whole. Then, of course, it took several more years for me to become proficient at it! I'm still learning.

As its name implies, DBT is primarily a behavioral treatment and, as such, places a high degree of emphasis on understanding and treating problems from a behavioral perspective. In practice, this means that the therapist strives to assess, observe, and describe behavior without "adding on" (e.g., interpretations, assumptions, "unconscious" drives or motivations) and offers specific solutions that are hypothesized to have the broadest impact on subsequent patterns of behavior. The behavioral chain analysis is the primary mode of assessment in DBT. Its role in the treatment cannot be overstated.

My goal in this book is to improve clinicians' mastery of this complex piece of DBT, and to see how it fits into the larger whole. When teaching a new skill in DBT, a therapist focuses on three levels of learning: acquisition, strengthening, and generalization. In this book, I offer the basics of chain analyses and how they are used in DBT. I also offer tips for strengthening one's knowledge and application of chain analyses so that a therapist can move from doing chain analyses in a rigid or rote manner to a more flexible approach that never loses sight of the core mission. Finally, I attempt to help therapists learn to generalize the chain analysis skill to multiple targets and situations. Throughout these processes, I also hope to dispel some myths about chain analyses related to what they are, when they should occur, and the style with which they should be conducted. I use many clinical examples throughout the book to illustrate the principles. These examples are composites of real cases that I, or my students, have seen over the past several years, modified to protect the clients' identities.

This book was several years in the making, and I have many people to thank and acknowledge for their important role in its creation. All of my mentors, and specifically Marsha Linehan, Ruth Striegel-Moore, Christy Telch, and Patricia Resick, have taught me what it means to be a clinical psychologist and scientist and have served as spectacular personal and professional role models. My students at the Dialectical Therapy Clinic at Rutgers, The State University of New Jersey, have also taught me how to be a more effective instructor and supervisor. The 2017–2018 cohort reviewed every chapter and gave detailed feedback, helping to shape it into its current form. For that, I thank Nikki Eskenasi, Kiki Fehling, Denise Guarino, Alex Hittman, Christopher Hughes, Alex King, Christine Laurine, Binh-an Nguyen, and Molly St. Denis. Two former students, William Buerger and Amanda Carson Wong, also provided rich clinical material that helped to form examples in this book. Nikki Eskenasi went the extra mile by helping me with all the figures and editing. This book would also not have come to fruition if it weren't for the constant enthusiasm of my dear editor, Kitty Moore ("Everyone should be doing chains!"), and Carolyn Graham at The Guilford Press.

I would also like to acknowledge my DBT co-trainers from over the years who have definitely influenced how I thought about the treatment and how I teach it to clinicians with a wide range of experiences and backgrounds. Charlie Swenson is a dear friend and colleague who, aside from Marsha, has taught me the most about DBT. I hear his voice as I write and therefore I know that he too is in this book. Lorie Ritschel, with whom I wrote an earlier article on chain analysis and conducted workshops on the topic, is a constant source of humor, clarity, and precision. I have also conducted workshops and trainings with Linda Dimeff, Elizabeth Simpson, Randy Wolbert, Alec Miller, Adam Payne, Sarah Reynolds, Jennifer Sayrs, and Tony DuBose, among others, and each of them has shaped me into a better teacher.

The year in which this book was finished also coincided with my participation in a Women in STEM leadership program at Rutgers. I am grateful for the university and Next Level Leadership for that program and specifically to Phoebe Atkinson, who served as my coach for the year, and my peers Grace Brannigan and Anne Piehl all of whom helped me stay on track with this book while offering never-ending support and care.

Finally, I would like to thank my husband, two boys, and two cats, who are a welcome respite from thinking about chains all the time.

Contents

CHAPTER 1

The Basics of the Chain Analysis

Barbara was a client whom I saw for therapy more than 15 years ago and yet I frequently think about her treatment and the lessons I learned from it. She was quite possibly the most difficult client I have ever treated (and I have seen some difficult clients!). There were challenges present in every session as well as the intransigence of the behaviors for which she came in seeking help. Barbara went through more than a year of dialectical behavior therapy (DBT) with little progress on her target behaviors and goals. Throughout the year, she frequently asked me if I had "figured out" her problems yet. There was an air of antagonism in her questions, which I resented and which likely interfered with both of our effectiveness in treatment. At the final session, she told me that she would write her problem on a piece of paper that I was not allowed to look at until after she left. On that paper, she had written "body dysmorphic disorder" (BDD). Despite working with her closely for a long stretch of time, I had no clue that BDD was a problem for her.

Similarly, Chet progressed through 5 months of a time-limited course of DBT before telling me about a critical aspect of his self-harming behavior. He had experienced so much shame about the fact that there was a sexual element to his behavior that he had never told anyone about it previously, despite having self-injured for more than 10 years and having had an extensive treatment history. In one of our final sessions, he told me that he had been leaving out a key detail in all our discussions about the factors involved in his self-injury behavior. When he finally revealed that he derived sexual pleasure from his self-injury, we did not have time to address this issue before he terminated.

In both cases, the lingering questions that remain with me are not "Why didn't they tell me sooner?" or "Why were they 'sabotaging' their treatment?" Instead, I wonder what questions I could have asked that would have yielded the needed information. How could I have improved my understanding of the problems they were experiencing? As a novice therapist for Barbara, I could have blamed it on inexperience. But I had worked with many clients by the time I met with Chet, which tells me that these issues are not only faced by new therapists. Instead, I think these situations tell us the critical importance of the role of assessment in treatment—its value cannot be understated. Accurate and thorough assessment is needed to change intransigent behavior, to generate effective solutions, and to move therapy forward toward the clients' goals. Yet, few clinicians are adequately trained in assessment or they incorrectly think about assessment as a phase to be gotten through at the start of treatment before the "meat" of therapy can occur. This book is an attempt to highlight the importance and necessity of assessment throughout treatment by explaining the purpose and procedure of chain analysis, the core assessment strategy in DBT.

I was fortunate to get my therapeutic training under the mentorship of Marsha Linehan, the founder of DBT. Given my immersion in DBT, the principles and strategies of DBT inform every intervention I do, even when I'm using another cognitive-behavioral therapy (CBT) protocol. One key aspect of DBT that informs my work in any modality is the critical value of assessment. As Linehan (1993) writes in the DBT manual, "Many, if not most, therapeutic errors are assessment errors; that is, they are therapeutic responses based on faulty understanding and assessment of the problem at hand" (p. 254). Assessment, therefore, is the foundation of effective treatment. Learning how to assess effectively involves knowing what questions to ask to get the most relevant information, what questions to avoid asking, and knowing when enough information has been obtained to move forward. These aspects of assessment can be taught in a systematic way, and this book will provide training in assessment, although more can always be gained through intensive trainings, workshops, literature reviews, and so forth.

DBT therapists use a chain analysis to gain a complete understanding of each single occurrence of a target behavior. Multiple chain analyses on the problem behavior are usually done over time, thereby adding information and revealing patterns. Although understanding the behavior is not sufficient for behavior change to occur, it is the underpinning for subsequent solution generation. For example, a client and therapist might be completely aware of all the factors that lead up to drinking episodes and their consequences, both negative and positive. However, without the client's motivation or interest in changing, the behavior is not going to change just by understanding the sequences of events. However, if there is interest in changing the behavior, identifying the critical controlling variables of the behavior is key. The chain analysis plays a critical role in case formulation and treatment planning in the earliest stage of treatment and continues to play a critical role throughout treatment as a means to understanding and treating behavior.

The essence of the chain analysis is to carefully assess the sequence of events leading to a behavior and the subsequent consequences. While the urge might be to do this in a narrative, open-ended format (e.g., "Describe to me what happened the night you used drugs"), DBT specifies five components of the chain that help to structure the assessment. These components are vulnerability factors, prompting event, links, problem behavior, and consequences. These are the nuts and bolts of chain analysis. In this chapter, I describe each of these components in detail, highlight some common mistakes made in assessing them, and provide examples of chains for a variety of different problem behaviors. The rest of the book will cover more complex issues as they relate to conducting chains in treatment.

COMPONENTS OF THE CHAIN ANALYSIS
- Vulnerability factors
- Prompting event
- Links (thought, emotion, behavior, other events of self and others)
- Target behavior
- Consequences (short term and long term)

The Five Components of Chain Analysis

The primary goal of any single chain analysis is to get an exceptionally clear description of the chain of events leading up to a single instance of a target behavior and the consequences that followed that particular occurrence. This goal usually requires a significant amount of orientation ahead of time for both the client and the therapist since this is not generally how our minds work or how many people think therapy should go. Instead, people generally want to "tell stories" about something that happened, not necessarily in a linear fashion, and focus on elements that they believe to be important, regardless of their actual importance in contributing to the target behavior. The chain analysis provides a structure to the assessment that aids the therapist and client in obtaining the relevant information to understanding the causes and maintaining the factors of a target behavior.

Figure 1.1 represents a visual cue for the chain analysis. The five components are chained together in the chronological sequence of an incident. I often have this visual in my mind as I assess because it keeps me on task and aware of what I need to do. Sharing the visual with clients is also incredibly important so that they are oriented to the procedure. In fact, Linehan included chain analysis as a skill to be taught to clients in the second edition of her skills manual (Linehan, 2015). In those materials, the visual links are present.

Target Behavior

The process of conducting a chain analysis typically follows a different sequence than the incident's chronology. The most important first step is a clear definition of the problem behavior, or *target behavior*, that occurred in that instance. It provides the foundation of the entire chain both topically and stylistically. I generally prefer the term "target behavior" because the client may not always concur that the behavior under analysis is a problem. In addition, a chain analysis can be done on the occurrence of any behavior, even those that have been effective in achieving desired goals, in order to better understand them.

In coming up with a description of the target behavior, it is necessary to provide specific details of the behavior. We call this the "topography of the behavior," by which we mean the form or "look" of the behavior, which needs to be put into concrete, behaviorally specific terms. For example, it is not sufficient for the behavior to be labeled as "self-injury" or "drug use." Instead, the therapist should zero in on eliciting specific details from the client in order to "see the behavior in her mind's eye." For example, "self-injury" could be "cut myself on my inner thigh with a shaving razor one time; the cut was about 2 inches long and bled a little; the cut occurred within about 2 seconds," or it could be "banged

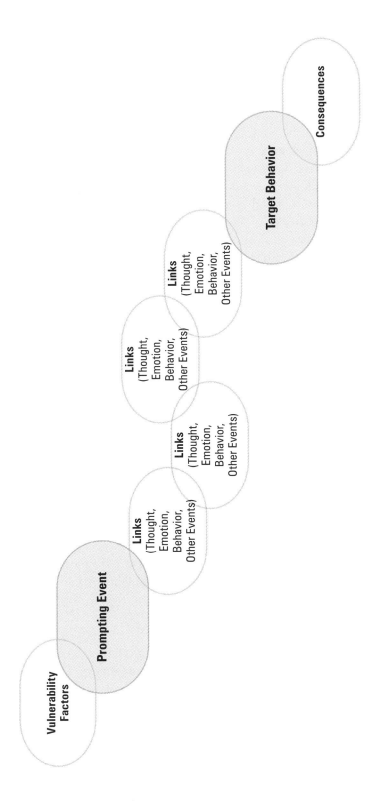

FIGURE 1.1. Chain analysis components.

my head against the concrete wall in my basement three times over the span of about a minute; felt significant pain but no bruising or bleeding occurred." Similarly, "drug use" can have many different topographies, and therefore specific details will help to fill in the picture: "I used intravenous heroin by shooting the needle in between my toes, approximately a fifth of a bag," or "I snorted three lines of cocaine along with drinking five shots of vodka over a period of 30 minutes."

Sometimes a target behavior can actually be a sequence of behaviors or a highly repetitive behavior over time. For example, a client reports that he repeatedly called his ex-girlfriend 50 times over the course of an hour. Or a client with trichotillomania describes an "episode" of hair pulling that lasts a total of 20 minutes. In such cases, it is usually helpful to treat the whole episode as the target behavior (i.e., "the episode of hair-pulling behavior that lasted 20 minutes, during which time the client repeatedly pulled hairs from the back of her head while sitting in front of her computer in her bedroom").

For some therapists, this line of questioning may initially feel too much like an interrogation in demanding the revelation of too many gruesome details, especially when the client is expressing a great deal of shame about the behavior or otherwise wants to gloss over it. The therapist may experience him- or herself as voyeuristic or insensitive. On the contrary, there are generally more occasions when therapists do not get enough details at the start of the chain and later find that it is harder to come back to get the particulars of what started the chain of behaviors as other details are filled in. Adopting a nonjudgmental stance in the assessment of the problem behavior (and throughout treatment) will likely help in reducing shame so that the therapist and client can talk about the behavior openly and clearly. Thorough orientation to the process, which is discussed in Chapter 2, is also immensely helpful here.

Prompting Event

Once the target behavior is clearly defined and behaviorally described, a therapist faces a decision point about where to go next. There is no "right" answer. However, I suggest therapists next address the *prompting event*. This is what I teach my new DBT clinicians to do. The "prompting event" is the event that appears to have been the precipitant (or "spark") for the target behavior. Often I describe it as "the event, that were it not to have occurred, the problem behavior would not have occurred." Like the problem behavior, it is important to anchor this event to a particular point in time; this helps in getting clear time points for the chain of events.

A client may identify a fight with his spouse at approximately 9:30 P.M. as the prompting event for a self-injurious episode that occurred around 11:45 P.M. Or a client may state that the prompting event for a 6:30 P.M. drinking episode was walking by a bar 5 minutes prior. Another client may state that waking up from a nightmare at 4:45 A.M. "set the stage" for an argument that got physical with her boyfriend at 8:00 P.M. that night. Each of these examples describes different scenarios in which the length of time between prompting event and problem behavior varies considerably. What should be evident by this is that the number of links between the two events can also vary substantially and that there is no predetermined rule for an appropriate length of time between the two.

That said, it is very important for the therapist to work with the client to identify the prompting event that is most relevant to the situation at hand. For example, a client may say that the prompting event for a self-injury episode on Friday was being fired from his job on the previous Tuesday. While it is likely valid that the job loss was an influential factor in the self-injury, an astute therapist would want to know what was different about Friday as opposed to Tuesday, Wednesday, or Thursday. Clearly, there must have been other events that increased the likelihood that self-injury would occur on Friday. These other events are important to assess and label because events closer in time to a behavior often exert more influence over the occurrence of the behavior. Therefore, zero-in on events that are more proximal in time to the target behavior. This will likely be more helpful in determining the controlling variables of the behavior and thus lead to more effective solution generation.

> To identify the prompting event, zero-in on events that are more proximal in time to the target behavior.

Another tricky aspect to determining a prompting event is when the client has difficulty identifying *one* discrete event and instead lists a multitude of factors that might have impacted the situation. For example, when asked what led to impulsive sexual behavior Sunday evening, the client might state, "I had a terrible day, starting with a flat tire on my way to church, which made me miss the service as well as spend money I didn't have to get the tire fixed. When I called my mother to tell her about it, she said, "These things always happen to you, you probably weren't being careful with your driving,' which made me feel crummy. And it was raining, so my friend canceled our plans to take a walk together and instead I just spent hours watching TV feeling bad for myself." When faced with this stream of events, it may be difficult to pinpoint *the* specific prompting event.

There are two possible paths to take to address this situation. One is to move away from the label of prompting event and instead just assess the sequence of events. You find out what happened first, what happened next, what happened after that, and so forth, until the chain of events is completed and the therapist has obtained a very clear idea of how the problem behavior of impulsive sex occurred. This turns the chain analyses away from becoming an overly academic exercise in which the therapist may lose the forest for the trees to come to the point in which a single prompting event is identified.

The other path to take is to try to isolate a single prompting event by engaging in hypothesis testing with the client. For example, in the scenario above, the therapist could change the variables to test out whether the target behavior would still have occurred (as best the client can guess). The therapist might ask, "Do you think had you not gotten the flat tire but still had a negative interaction with your mom and canceled the date with your friend, that you would have had impulsive sex?" or "Do you think that had you made it out with your friend after the flat tire and interaction with your mom, that you still would have had impulsive sex?" Often, through these lines of questioning, the client can provide information that highlights an event that was more critical than the others in terms of its impact on subsequent problem behaviors.

There are advantages to each approach to determining the prompting event. In general, in early chains between a therapist just getting to know a client, I am more likely to suggest the first approach. That is, just assessing the sequence of events rather than getting bogged down trying to find a specific, sole prompting event helps move assessment along. However, in future chains, especially when a behavior isn't changing despite attempts to intervene, there might be an indication that a more fine-grained assessment is needed (see Chapter 6). In such cases, getting really clear on what constituted the prompting event might be an important unsolved piece of the puzzle.

In the case of habitual behaviors, it can be difficult to isolate a prompting event. With a behavior that occurs daily or multiple times a day (e.g., skin picking or drinking/drug use for some clients), there is often no specific prompting event since the behavior is likely to occur no matter what. This would be similar to trying to find the prompting event for me taking a shower today. The prompt is likely just waking up and having it be a new day! However, given the importance of focusing on variables more proximal in time to the problem behavior and the reliance on a structure in conducting a chain, it is still important to identify something as a starting point of the chain. Often, starting with when the individual first thought about engaging in the problem behavior could be an anchor.

A last critical point is to understand that a prompting event can be external to the client (an event in the environment or another person's behavior) or internal (a thought, a nightmare). The latter is more likely to be the identified prompting event when the client cannot name a particular precipitant to the thought. For example, the client might say, "I had a flashback of my rape just totally out of the blue and that led me to use drugs." For the purposes of analyzing the drug use episode, this assessment of the prompting event would likely be sufficient, although it is very likely that there was an antecedent to the flashback and that identification of this antecedent might itself be a very important target in treatment. However, if the client describes the prompting event as something like "I just suddenly thought that I was totally alone in the world and that set off the chain toward self-injury," the therapist would likely want to assess what led to that thought since that thought might be a modifiable link in the chain. For example, the client might then say that this thought occurred after a friend failed to respond to her text message. We might then label the lack of response by the friend (within 15 minutes of sending the text) as the prompting event, which was followed by the client's *interpretation* that she was totally alone. Framing it in this way might also lead the client to recognize how the links are related and how the thought did not come "out of the blue" and in fact was caused by a notable event.

Vulnerability Factors

Once the target behavior and prompting event have been identified, a next area to explore is the client's *vulnerability factors*. "Vulnerability factors" refer to variables that may have made the client more susceptible to the effects of the prompting event *in that particular instance*. A helpful way to think about vulnerability factors is to consider those events, situations, thoughts, or states of mind that make a person more likely to experience emotion dysregulation. These can include poor sleep, poor eating, physical illness, and not taking medications as prescribed on that particular day. Vulnerability factors could also consist of other recent life events that have accumulated to make the client feel overwhelmed or taxed. As in the example above, a job loss a few days prior along with the ensuing feelings and worries related to a difficult situation would likely make the client more vulnerable to a negative event (prompting event) that happened on the day of the self-injury. Vulnerability factors often address the question of "what made the target behavior more likely to occur on that particular day (or at that particular time)," especially when the prompting event occurs frequently in the client's life. For example, a client might identify a fight with her boyfriend as the prompting event leading to self-injury later that evening. However, the therapist may well be aware that fights with the boyfriend are a frequent occurrence and self-injury does not occur at the same frequency level. To identify vulnerability factors, the therapist may ask, "Was there anything that made you more vulnerable to the effects of this fight on this day?"

There are two common problems that I have seen come up repeatedly in the assessment of vulnerability factors. One is when the client (or therapist) identifies too many factors to be helpful. Many clients with multiple problems who meet criteria for a number of psychological disorders will readily identify a host of problems related to the regulation of sleep, medication, eating, exercise, and so forth, all of which may impact their vulnerability to being in emotion mind. While it may be true that these factors contribute to the overall chaos, stress, and problems in clients' lives, they are likely not all directly relevant to the assessment of the specific problem behavior. Thus, the therapist needs to stay mindful to the task of the chain analysis, which is really to home-in on this one specific episode. At the risk of being redundant, I want to stress the importance of this: the therapist has to constantly be asking him- or herself "Why did *this* occur on *this* specific day?" If the client always (or often) has dysregulated sleep but does not always engage in binge drinking, then dysregulated sleep although likely not *helpful* is also likely not a primary controlling variable of the drinking.

> To identify vulnerability factors, ask, Why did this behavior occur on this specific day?

The second problem is when the therapist or client labels a long-standing problem as a vulnerability factor. For example, I have often seen therapists identifying "a diagnosis of borderline personality disorder" (BPD) as a vulnerability factor. Here it is important to validate that yes, a person with BPD is likely more vulnerable than someone without BPD to the effects of various emotional stimuli (this forms the basis for the biosocial theory of DBT; Linehan, 1993). However, between-person vulnerability factors are not really relevant to the chain. Instead, within-person factors are important. We assume that a person with a diagnosis of BPD has BPD-like behaviors and vulnerabilities on a regular basis. What made her *more* vulnerable to the prompting event *on that day?*

Links

Moving along in the sequence of events of a chain, I now typically turn to *links*. The "links" of the chain refer to any events, private or overt, that lead the client from the prompting event to the target behavior. These links may include cognitions, emotions, urges, interpersonal events, other external events, secondary target behaviors, and others. Secondary targets, also known as "dialectical dilemmas," refer to patterns of behavior that interfere with the successful treatment of primary target behaviors (see Linehan, 1993, for rich clinical descriptions of these behavioral patterns and their role in maintaining target behaviors). In assessing the links, it is important for the therapist to recognize that not every single link between prompting event and target behavior is necessarily dysfunctional or problematic. In fact, there are often many functional links in the chain in which the client behaved effectively or normatively. The nonjudgmental stance here remains important since the therapist is just wondering what occurred between Point A and Point B, not necessarily what all the problematic things the client did were.

Questions to assess links include "What happened next?"; "How did you get from X to Y?"; "What thoughts were you having here?"; "What emotions or feelings were you having?"; and so on. As I point out in Chapter 2, there is tremendous value to both the therapist and the client in visually writing out the links in the chain on a whiteboard or easel as they are being discussed. This strategy is especially useful when assessing links because it calls the sequence of events into view. In assessing links, the therapist wants the sequence to make sense and not have gaping holes in the chain.

Depending on how much time elapsed between the prompting event and the behavior, assessment of these links can take a little or a lot of time. Different problems emerge based on this time gap. When there is very little time that elapsed, a client may be quick to say, "I just did it," without recognizing the presence of any thoughts or emotions or urges. Slowing down this moment in time and doing an extreme microanalysis may be useful in these situations. For example, clients might say something like "All of a sudden, the razor was in my hand," as though some magical process was involved. In such cases, the therapist would want to ask a lot of detailed questions about what the client was thinking, feeling, and doing in the moments, or seconds, leading up to that point. Once the client knows that this level of detail is desired, it might be easier to obtain information about links in future chains because clients are made more aware of the sequence of events.

Conversely, a person may describe in detail what happened during the *hours* leading up to the problem behavior. Taking the time to analyze each link in such a situation would take much more time than a single therapy session affords. In these instances, the therapist may have to zero-in on the most relevant factors. Obviously the most relevant factors are not necessarily known to the therapist from the beginning, so this is not always an easy task. What is often most helpful for me to remember is that I need to see in my own mind how the client got from Point A to Point B. If details are too fuzzy, or if I have to make too many assumptions, to get that picture in my mind, then I need to collaboratively assess more. At other times, I may have to cut the client off in order to move along the sequence of time in order to get information that helps me understand how the behavior occurred.

Given that DBT was designed to address how emotions drive behavior, the therapist also wants to focus specifically on emotions in the links of the chain analysis. That is, a therapist should not consider a chain complete unless he or she knows about the presence and intensity of emotions along the sequence of events. The therapist also does not want to assume that a client can adequately label his or her emotional experiences (at least in the early stages of therapy). There are lots of reasons why a client may not know how to label emotional experiences adequately. A client may label every feeling as "upset" without knowing the specific emotions. Or a client may label every unpleasant experience as "anger" because that is what seems most salient and notable. Thus, the clinician has to work with the client to parse different emotional experiences and learn to label them accurately in order to most effectively approach them. Again, if it doesn't make sense to me, it's a cue to follow up with additional inquiry ("How is it that you felt shame when you didn't receive a text back from your friend?").

Ultimately, you want the links to tell the story with just enough detail to have a clear, clinically rich picture of how the sequence unfolded. You have probably noticed by now that this process is not intended to be so exhaustive that you cover every single second between prompting event and target behavior. To assess to that level of specificity would likely take more time than the sequence of events themselves. It would also likely exhaust both the client and the therapist! Thus, with practice, you want to find the "sweet spot" of enough detail without scrutinizing the minutiae of each moment.

Consequences

Last, but certainly not least, a therapist wants to assess the *consequences* of the problem behavior. Typically, the function of assessing consequences is to determine whether there were any contingencies that function as reinforcers, and thus make it more likely for the behavior to occur again in the future. However, this is often not how the term "consequences" is interpreted by the client. If the therapist were to ask, "What were the consequences of you pushing your sister during that fight?," the client might respond, "I felt awful and I fear that our relationship will never be the same again." However, when pressed to answer "Immediately after you pushed her, what happened both within you and also with your sister?," the client might respond, "I felt momentarily really powerful and my sister backed down." While the long-term consequences are considered more important by the client, the short-term reinforcing consequences make it more likely that she will push her sister (or someone else) in similar circumstances in the future. Some recognition of this and relevant solution generation will be needed in order to address this obstacle to improvement. Thus, it is vital that the therapist assess immediate consequences to the behavior in addition to longer-term consequences. It is also incredibly important to note that most of the time, we are not aware of the effects of contingencies on our behavior. Assessing immediate consequences will increase awareness of these factors and identify factors that might be modifiable with some effort.

Together, these five components form the basis of the chain analyses. The links that constitute the completed chain can range from five to hundreds depending on the amount of time covered and the complexity of the situation. It can take 3 minutes to several hours to complete a chain analysis depending on a different set of factors. In other words, it's complicated! As always, a clear focus on the principles and function of the chain are important:

1. Remember that the primary function of chain analysis is to assess a single occurrence of a target behavior *in order to* most effectively generate solutions that will impact the occurrence of that behavior in the future.

2. Identifying the critical controlling variables is key to this mission.

3. Remember to avoid assumptions and instead rely on your own wise mind to obtain an understanding of how one link leads to another (and another, and another, . . .).

Below are three representative examples highlighting chains that come from three target categories in DBT: life-threatening behavior (contemplating jumping from the edge of a roof), therapy-interfering behavior (yelling in group at other group members), and quality-of-life interfering behavior (shoplifting). They cover a range of timeframes from 5 minutes to a few hours. They each highlight various types of links and include a focus on emotion. In future examples, I use dialogue to indicate how a therapist might assess specifically for these components. However, here I just describe the components of the chain. Accompanying each description of the chain analysis in text form is a visual illustration of the chain using the model in Figure 1.1. Things to note throughout are the level of behavioral specificity involved in detailing each component and the fact that it "makes sense" to naïve readers, even without knowing more details or history about the client. Hopefully, they all illustrate how different points of intervention can be identified along the sequence of events.

Examples of Chain Analyses

Chain Analysis of an Incident of Suicidal Behavior

Target behavior: Went to roof of six-story parking garage at 2:30 A.M. Sunday morning, dangled feet over edge, thought about jumping ("If I were to jump right now, I would show everyone how awful my life is and I would end my suffering"). Sat there for approximately 30 minutes, ruminating about suicide.

Prompting event: At boyfriend's house with several of his friends over to play a video game. At approximately 11:00 P.M., I asked him a question ("Can I play this game with you?") and he ignored me.

Vulnerability factors: Boyfriend and I were together since about 5:00 P.M. His friends came over around 7:00 P.M. and they were loud and obnoxious with each other and I felt left out. This feeling got progressively worse until the moment that I asked him if I could join the video game they were playing.

Links: Over the course of about 3½ hours:

- Silence from boyfriend in response to my question. He keeps talking to his friends.
- Thought: I feel so humiliated.
- Emotion: Shame, humilation.
- Thought: What a jerk! How can he do this to me?
- Emotion: Anger.
- Thought: I could just disappear and he wouldn't even notice. I'm so useless. [secondary target: self-invalidation]
- Behavior: Went upstairs to bedroom, laid on bed, watched TV on and off for a couple hours, and fell asleep for a bit.
- Thought: He hasn't even noticed or cared that I'm gone.
- Emotions: Anger, sadness.
- Behavior: Went back downstairs, said, "What's happening?"
- Event: Boyfriend and friends said, "Not much," continued to focus on video game.
- Behavior: Went into kitchen, sat at table, drank two beers, and ruminated (approximately 1:00–1:30 A.M.).
- Emotions: Anger, sadness (intensifying).
- Thought: He wouldn't even care if I killed myself.
- Behavior: Started crying.
- Thought: I should just do it [kill myself].

- Thought: I should call my therapist but it's late and I don't want to wake her.
- Behavior: Drank two more beers (approximately 1:45–2:15 A.M.).
- Thought: I'm just going to do it. I'm just going to kill myself.
- Emotions: Excitement?
- Behavior: Left out of back door, slammed door, walked three blocks to parking garage, took elevator to roof.
- Thought: I can do this; it will show him.
- Behavior: Walked to edge, sat down.

Consequences:

- Immediate: Felt a bit of a "rush" sitting there but also extreme anxiety, almost panic, quickly set in. I thought, "I don't have the guts to do this."
- Texted boyfriend where I was. He immediately texted back and told me to come straight home.
- I went home and he yelled at me, telling me that I should never do that again. His friends left and we spent some time in bed watching TV together before we both fell asleep.
- Emotions: Calm, relieved.

Commentary: This chain (illustrated in Figure 1.2) describes an event that covers the span of several hours. The essence here is to make sure that enough detail is captured that one can see the chain and understand how each link is connected. In reading the chain, you can see how these events happen even if you also see all the opportunities for things to have gone differently, or all the missed opportunities to act more effectively. Careful attention is paid to thoughts, emotions, and behaviors of both the client and others.

Chain Analysis of "Acting Out" in Group

Target behavior: Yelled, "I shouldn't be in this group—you all have more problems than me!" in group around 6:45 P.M. (group is held from 6:00 to 8:00 P.M.).

Prompting event: The group leader asked who wanted to share their homework (around 6:10 P.M.).

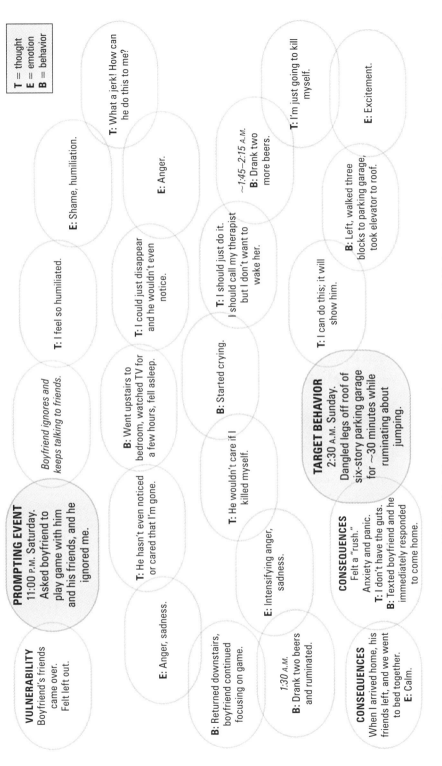

T = thought
E = emotion
B = behavior

VULNERABILITY
Boyfriend's friends came over. Felt left out.

PROMPTING EVENT
11:00 P.M. Saturday. Asked boyfriend to play game with him and his friends, and he ignored me.

Boyfriend ignores and keeps talking to friends.

T: I feel so humiliated.

E: Shame, humiliation.

T: What a jerk! How can he do this to me?

E: Anger.

E: Anger, sadness.

T: He hasn't even noticed or cared that I'm gone.

B: Went upstairs to bedroom, watched TV for a few hours, fell asleep.

T: I could just disappear and he wouldn't even notice.

T: I should just do it. I should call my therapist but I don't want to wake her.

~1:45–2:15 A.M.
B: Drank two more beers.

T: I'm just going to kill myself.

E: Excitement.

E: Intensifying anger, sadness.

T: He wouldn't care if I killed myself.

B: Started crying.

T: I can do this; it will show him.

B: Left, walked three blocks to parking garage, took elevator to roof.

B: Returned downstairs, boyfriend continued focusing on game.

1:30 A.M.
B: Drank two beers and ruminated.

TARGET BEHAVIOR
2:30 A.M. Sunday. Dangled legs off roof of six-story parking garage for ~30 minutes while ruminating about jumping.

CONSEQUENCES
Felt a "rush."
Anxiety and panic.
T: I don't have the guts.
B: Texted boyfriend and he immediately responded to come home.

CONSEQUENCES
When I arrived home, his friends left, and we went to bed together.
E: Calm.

FIGURE 1.2. Chain analysis of an incident of suicidal behavior.

17

Vulnerability: Slept only 1 hour the night before, had very stressful day at work, did not want to go to skills group because I wanted to go home and sleep instead.

Links:

- Behavior: I looked around and noticed that I was the only one that had my homework sheet completed.
- Thought: What assholes! Am I the only one here who cares about getting better?
- Emotion: Irritability.
- Event: Group leader starts asking another member about "what got in the way" of homework this week.
- Behavior: "Zoned out"; stopped listening and ruminated about my desire for sleep.
- Event: Co-leader nudged me and whispered for me to stay present.
- Emotion: Shame, anger.
- Thought: Why is she bugging me? She should get everyone else in line.
- Event: Group leader goes to another person and asks the same question.
- Thought: This is bullshit. Total waste of my time. I could be sleeping right now.
- Emotion: Anger.
- Feeling: Intense fatigue.
- Event: Leader gets to me and asks me about my homework.
- Behavior: I tell her about my use of mindfulness skills this week.
- Event: She tells me that I didn't do it quite right and starts correcting me.
- Emotion: Intense shame and anger.
- Don't remember thoughts before yelling.

Consequences:

- Co-leader asked me to step out of group. I grabbed all my things and just left. Intense anger.

- Went outside, smoked cigarette (relief from stress), got in car, and sped home.
- Knew I would "get shit" about this from my individual therapist later. Felt angry and guilty.

Commentary: This chain of events (illustrated in Figure 1.3) occurred over a shorter period of time, about 45 minutes. A similar focus on detailing thoughts, feelings, and behaviors is present. Note the specificity of description throughout as well.

Chain Analysis of Stealing Behavior

Target behavior: In department store, stole three scarves by placing them in my bag and walking out of the store unnoticed. Friday, approximately 5:00 P.M.

Prompting event: Noticed a store clerk looking at me (approximately 4:55 P.M.).

Vulnerability factors: Had felt depressed and down all day; had done nothing but lay in bed while on the Internet for hours. Finally got self to get up and activate by going to the mall but still felt depressed and lonely.

Links: Over the course of about 5 minutes:

- Thought: She's suspicious of me. She thinks I'm going to steal something just because I'm black.
- Emotion: Anger.
- Thought: That bitch, I'll show her.
- Behavior: Walked around store looking for "easiest" thing to steal.
- Emotions: Excitement, anger.
- Behavior: Saw scarves and noticed there was no security tag on them.
- Thought: What dumbasses they are.
- Behavior: Looked around to see if any clerks were nearby.
- Thought: Now's the time to just do it.
- Emotion: Excitement, fear.

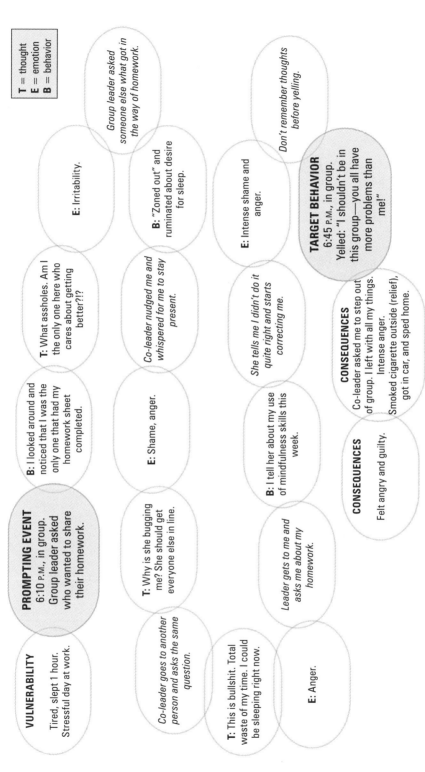

FIGURE 1.3. Chain analysis of acting out in group.

Consequences:

- Immediate: Excitement and relief from fear. Thought, I got away with it again!
- Quickly followed by thought of "I can't believe I did it again; I have no self-control," shame and disappointment.

Commentary: In this example (illustrated in Figure 1.4), the analysis covers a very short period of time, which is often the situation for more impulsive behaviors like this one. Even though the period of time is shorter, there is still careful attention to all of the components of the chain.

In this chapter, I laid the foundations for the chain analysis and provided a few examples of what an exhaustive chain might look like. I used relatively straightforward examples so that one could see how a sequential chain plays out, with each of the five components specified. However, in "real life," the assessment process is often multidimensional with unexpected issues frequently occurring that make it difficult to conduct chains in a straightforward and simple manner. Throughout the rest of this book, I cover a range of chain analyses that demonstrate their use throughout a variety of situations and complexities.

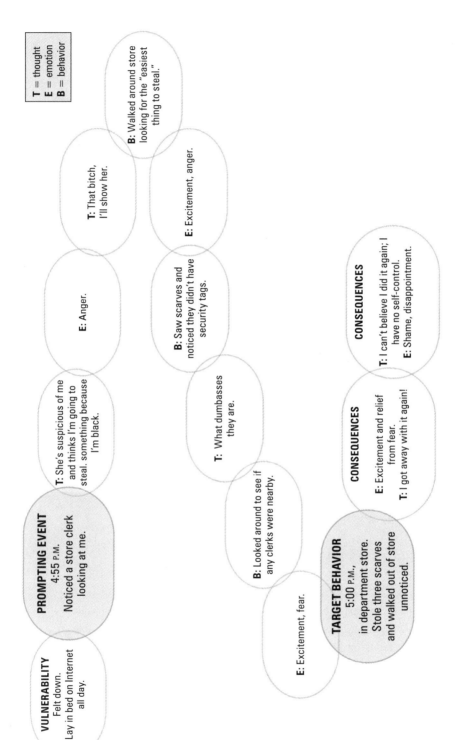

FIGURE 1.4. Chain analysis of stealing behavior.

CHAPTER 2

Guidelines for Client Orientation and Collaboration for Chain Analyses

I n this chapter, I discuss guidelines to follow when orienting clients to the procedures of chain analyses and for increasing collaboration. These guidelines will help make the process less technical and robotic and more lively and cooperative. Given its critical role in the conduct of the chain analysis, much of this chapter is devoted to the process of orienting clients to the rationale, process, and importance of chain analyses. The more successful a therapist is with this process, the greater the likelihood that the chains will be successful at obtaining the necessary information to make positive changes.

Orientation to Chain Analysis

The importance of orientation reflects a core value of DBT: the therapist is to be *transparent* as a clinician. This means that the therapist frequently describes what he or she is doing and why he or she is doing it. One of the assumptions about treatment in DBT is that the therapeutic relationship is a real relationship between equals (Linehan, 1993), and one of the ways in which that spirit is manifested is by the therapist operating as though the client can know everything that he or she knows about principles of behavior and behavior change. In essence, you want to help your clients to master the skill of analyzing their behavior as well as you have mastered it. This skill will help them to work toward solving their own problems independently (i.e., gradually becoming their own therapists). Examples of general orienting instructions will be given as well as illustrations as to how to handle difficult therapy situations. Also, I provide suggestions for different ways in which the chain analysis can be conducted that will increase the likelihood of success.

Why Orientation Is Important

Orienting means giving the client information about the purpose, process, and requirements of a task or procedure (see Linehan, 1993). In DBT, and behavior therapies more broadly, orientation is used at the beginning of therapy to give information about treatment as a whole, as well as any time a new procedure or assignment is generated. Specifically, Linehan (1993) states, "Before each instance of new learning, [an] orientation or task overview should be presented directly and deliberately to the patient in order to provide precise information about what has to be learned, as well as a clarification of the conceptual model within with the learning will take place" (p. 282). It is assumed that such orientation is necessary to have clients buy in to the task and thus increase their commitment to the task overall, which likely increases motivation to follow through.

> Orientation involves giving the client information about the purpose, process, and requirements of a task or procedure.

Clinicians are best served by explaining to clients what the chain analysis is, how it works, and what it is intended to do. Although there are some circumstances in which a therapist might quickly delve into a chain prior to telling the client about the procedure, these are the exceptions rather than the rule. For example, in a crisis situation early in treatment, when the therapist has to assess the level of risk associated with a recent suicide attempt, he or she might have to jump into a chain analysis of this attempt without spending time telling the client what exactly he or she is doing. However, in general, orienting the client to the chain analysis is vital in treatment.

A chain analysis will go better the more the client is personally invested in its success. What makes a client (or anyone, really) want to do a task? It is partly about knowing the rationale for the task. I know that my motivation to engage in any task is significantly affected by whether

I believe it is meaningful and important. Like most people, I tend to put off tasks that don't hold much value for me. We can't expect clients to jump on board to do a chain analysis if they don't understand why they're being asked to do it or how it might benefit them. They might go through the motions of answering questions but without a sense of purpose, and they will be less invested and interested in the outcome. I have often seen novice clinicians jump into doing a chain without first telling the person *what* they were doing and *why* they were doing it. What follows then is more likely to be a noncollaborative venture that yields less valuable information or it will be a confusing jumble of information because the client doesn't understand what the therapist was trying to do.

How to Orient Clients to Chain Analysis

It is important to use the label "chain analysis" early in treatment. This labeling has many benefits. One, it increases the transparency of the process and creates a shared language. Two, it communicates to the client that you have a clear strategy with a particular goal in mind. Three, if you use the term early in treatment, you avoid having to explain it over and over again. For example, in a later session, you can say, "So of course we need to do a chain on that behavior," and the client will immediately know what the process looks like and what it's intended to do.

The following is an example of what an orientation to the chain analysis could look like the first time it is used in treatment:

> "In some ways, it is so great that you had this experience this week, because that gives me the opportunity to orient you to an important part of this treatment. It's called the 'chain analysis.' Have you heard of that before? [If yes, discuss client's previous understanding of this strategy and correct any misconceptions.] The chain analysis is a step-by-step picture of all the events, thoughts, and feelings leading up to this target behavior, as well as the consequences of the behavior. It needs to be pretty detailed and really tries to focus in on the exact sequence of events as they occurred in those moments.
>
> "The reason we do chain analyses in DBT is to get a complete understanding of all the potential contributors to this behavior so that we can figure out what needs to change in order to get this behavior to stop. At times it might feel like I'm being really particular or overly detailed. I want you to tell me when you feel that way

and I also want you to know why I'm doing it. The first few times we do one, it may take a bit of time but once we get the hang of doing them together, it will likely go a lot faster. How does this all sound to you?"

In this brief example, there are a number of salient points to note for effectively orienting clients to chain analysis. First, the therapist very explicitly used the term "chain analysis," which provides a common term to be used in future interactions, and satisfies the need for transparency. It also provides a clear definition of what a chain analysis entails. Clarity will help eliminate surprises, and the sense that the client does not know what is happening. In addition, it shows how the therapist is anticipating concerns that the client might raise, such as thinking the therapist is asking for too many details, and it highlights a problem-solving attitude about them. Finally, the therapist asks for feedback and commentary, which helps to reduce the sense that the client is being "lectured to." The task is not meant to be (or feel like) a chore. Thus, the therapist needs to present it in a way that highlights the utility of the process, not just relying on a "We have to do this because the manual says so" message. Once a clear orientation like this is provided, in future sessions the therapist can often cut straight to the chase without having to provide another explanation of the process.

Countering Client Avoidance

Ideally, the first experience of a chain analysis is positive for both therapist and client. For the therapist, the goals are to gain an understanding of the client's behavior and feel competent to suggest one or two viable solutions to implement. Clients need to feel they have gained an understanding of their own behavior, feel understood by the therapist, and feel optimistic about being able to take the steps needed to change the unwanted behavior. Making this first chain a positive experience will also increase the likelihood that the client will recognize the need for analyses in the future and willingly comply with the procedure. Of course, while therapists want the first chain to be a positive experience, they don't always work out that way. Especially early in treatment, when the therapist does not know the client very well, every move has the potential to hit a landmine. The risk is that the therapist might act overly cautious and prioritize positivity over the primary function of the chain. When this happens, the therapist could easily allow the client to dominate the direction of the chain or get off the chain altogether, which negates its purpose.

Let's continue with the scenario presented above in which the therapist has just finished orienting the client to the chain:

THERAPIST: OK, so let's get to work on doing a chain on your recent self-injury.

CLIENT: Do we have to? I really don't want to talk about it.

THERAPIST: Oh really? How come?

CLIENT: Well, it was a one-time thing. It's not going to be a problem anymore. Rehashing it will only make me feel worse.

THERAPIST: I'm really glad you believe this won't happen again. Do you think there is anything we can learn from what happened by discussing it?

CLIENT: No. I know that I'm not going to do it again this time.

THERAPIST: OK then, sounds like you are determined to not self-injure again, which is great. Let's move on to something else.

In this scenario, the therapist allows the client to control the agenda and avoid talking about the self-harm. While there may be validity in what the client is saying (in fact, it might be the very last time this client ever self-injures and it is likely that talking about it will increase negative emotions), the therapist colludes in avoidance of the topic. Returning to orientation and commitment will be important strategies for the therapist to utilize to increase engagement in the task.

Returning to this example, let's see how it might go a different way, with the client moving toward willingness to engage in the chain analysis.

THERAPIST: OK, so let's get to work on doing a chain on your recent self-injury.

CLIENT: Do we have to? I really don't want to talk about it.

THERAPIST: Oh really? How come?

CLIENT: Well, it was a one-time thing. It's not going to be a problem anymore. Rehashing it will only make me feel worse.

THERAPIST: Ah, I can see how you wouldn't want to engage in a chain analysis in that case. And I really hope that this episode was your very last self-injury ever. However, I think there can be a lot of value in doing a chain analysis, even in this circumstance. Can I tell you why I think that?

CLIENT: Sure.

THERAPIST: One reason is that it is still early in treatment and I don't know you that well. When we do a chain together, it helps me to see how your thoughts, emotions, and behaviors go together and I get a better understanding of who you are, even if this was a one-time event.

CLIENT: OK.

THERAPIST: Another reason is that even though your commitment to not self-injure again is strong right now, we all know that commitment to something can wax and wane and emotions certainly play a large role in that. So I want to figure out what went into you self-injuring this week in order to see what your vulnerabilities might be in the future. That way, we can shore up all your defenses and really be sure that you are in good shape to fight off urges if they occur again.

CLIENT: I guess that makes sense.

THERAPIST: And there's one last reason I can think of in this moment. Again, I don't know you very well but I'm guessing that you, like most people, want to avoid experiences that make you feel strong negative emotions. This makes complete and total sense of course! The downside to this desire to avoid, though, is that negative emotions are a natural part of life, and if we avoid talking about problems that cause them, we never learn how to effectively deal with them. In DBT, we are going to spend a lot of time talking about emotions, ways to manage them effectively, and ways to live with them. I would hate for us to start our treatment with me somehow giving you and your brain the message that we should avoid discussing difficult topics. So, are you with me?

CLIENT: Yeah, I guess so. It is true that I often tell people I don't want to work on things after-the-fact and then things never improve.

THERAPIST: Exactly! And I'm asking you to do this chain with me because I really want things to improve for you and I know that this is the way forward. I'm so glad you are willing to do it with me now.

TABLE 2.1. Some Reasons for Chain Analysis Early in Treatment

- It helps the therapist get to know the client better by seeing how the client's thoughts, emotions, and behaviors go together.
- It helps the client and the therapist see what contributed to the behavior and helps identify possible future vulnerabilities so they can be addressed.
- If the client avoids talking about problems that cause difficult emotions, he or she will never learn how to deal with them effectively.

In this scenario, the therapist uses a lot of validation to communicate what is normal and adaptive about what the client is expressing and feeling. There is also orientation to the reasons to do a chain analysis and a straightforward listing of these reasons. See Table 2.1 for a summary of the reasons from the above example. When a therapist is direct with the client, it can also bring a quality of "radical genuineness" to the interaction as it indicates that the client is capable of hearing what the therapist has to say and communicates that the therapist and client are equals in this partnership. Finally, the example highlights that the therapist finds immense value in the exercise personally and enthusiastically communicates that importance directly to the client. In so doing, he or she is promoting the significance of the process and thereby increasing the likelihood for collaboration and buy-in.

So far, the example describes the process of orientation to chain analysis when the therapist uses it for the first time in treatment. Orientation to these first chains has to be accompanied by a description of what chains are and why they are used. It is important that the therapist appear invested in the process and communicate enthusiasm about it given its role as the foundation to changing behavior in effective ways. Using clear and descriptive language, including terms such as "chain analysis," "target behavior," "prompting event," and the like, is necessary to increase collaboration.

Although orientation is a necessary and required part of DBT when a task is first presented, the strategy also proves quite useful in later sessions when there is a wavering of willingness to engage in the chain analysis. In these cases, the therapist might return to orienting from scratch again (if viewed as useful) or remind the client about the earlier orientation conversation. For example:

CLIENT: I really don't want to do a chain today. I hate them and I would rather talk about my roommate situation.

THERAPIST: I get that entirely. I wouldn't want to do something I hated either. I would much rather you love chain analyses because I do and I see them as so helpful. Do you remember what the reasons are for chains in DBT and why I insist on doing them with you?

CLIENT: Sort of. You want to know what led up to me hurting myself.

THERAPIST: Yes, but why do I want to do that?

CLIENT: I guess so we can figure out how I could have done things differently. I already know what I could have done differently; I just didn't do it!

THERAPIST: Ah, so maybe willfulness showed up? Or was it that you didn't think of what skillful things you could have done until afterward?

CLIENT: I don't know.

THERAPIST: OK, so this really highlights for me why we want to do this chain together. We really need to zero-in on this aspect specifically— what shows up that interferes with you acting more skillfully. Because I agree with you, we've talked about solutions before and I know you know the skills. But something is happening that gets in the way of you using them when you most need to. Will you work on this with me? If we get right into it, we'll likely have some time remaining for us to discuss your roommate problem

CLIENT: I'll try.

I'd like to make an important point here about how to think about a client's dislike of chains. A chain analysis is not meant to be overly aversive. Clients often view the analysis as solely intended to punish them for a problematic behavior. While it might be true that doing a chain analysis is an unpleasant experience for the client, if the therapist focuses too much on its function as a punisher (either unintentionally or with a mentality of the client "paying the price" of his or her behavior), the client will ultimately work to avoid it. In the best case scenario, the client will avoid it by not engaging in the problem behavior again. In fact, there are those rare instances in which a client will say "I thought about doing [problematic behavior] but didn't want to have to talk with you about it so I decided not to." However, in my experience, the more a therapist focuses on the punishing aspects of the chain, the more likely the client will avoid by lying about the behavior or saying he or she no longer wishes to change the behavior in question. Thus, the therapist has to walk a fine line—using the chain analysis as a negative consequence when that proves effective at reducing the behavior and also focusing extensively on the usefulness of the analysis regardless of whether the behavior was desired or not. The therapist will want to be careful not to convey the chain analysis as a chore to be endured but instead as a valuable learning experience for both the therapist and the client.

Much of this communication about the chain has to do with the therapist's own attitude about chains. Consider the following:

CLIENT: Do we really have to do a chain? You know I hate them.

THERAPIST: I know you do. But you self-injured this week, so now we have to.

In just this one sentence, the therapist communicated that chains are a mandatory consequence of "bad" behavior. The idea that "we have to" do a chain also conveys the notion that both the therapist and the client are somehow prisoners to the rules of DBT. This attitude models to the client an inflexibility about the process and negates the value of the chain. Imagine instead:

CLIENT: Do we really have to do a chain? You know I hate them.

THERAPIST: I know you do. And I hate that you hate them! Because they are so important and I really believe they will get us to your goals. So let's get to it!

Here, the therapist quickly conveys enthusiasm and the rationale for the chains while also acknowledging the client's feelings about them. Linking chain analyses to the client's goals for treatment and life can be a very useful motivator. The therapist also adopts a hopeful tone about the benefits of chains and dives right in rather than spending time debating their merits.

> Linking chain analyses to the client's goals for treatment and life can be a very useful motivator.

This last point is an especially important one when faced with a client who does not want to participate in a chain analysis. The reasons for client avoidance are many: experiencing extreme shame about the behavior and having to talk about it with the therapist; willfulness about either the task or a previously made commitment to stop the behavior; a desire to speak about other topics; a difficulty in describing events in a sequential manner (see below); or some combination of all of these. The client may indeed want to talk about the problem but by storytelling rather than by doing the process of the chain analysis. All of these factors are certainly understandable given the context, and yet each will likely interfere with gaining information in a systematic manner, which would be effective in subsequently generating solutions.

So how do you get a client on board with a chain analysis? As in the above example, the therapist gently elicits from the client the rationale for engaging in chains. Asking the client to explain will likely help with buy-in and also help to avoid the situation in which the therapist slips into lecturing the client ("This is good for you!") or conveying that he or she is held hostage by the treatment ("DBT says we have to do one")—for example: "Remember back when you started treatment, we talked about why we do chain analysis in DBT and what function they serve? Can you list for me now the reasons we do them?" The therapist can then help the client generate reasons if he or she no longer remembers or otherwise refuses. Next, the therapist can briefly assess what is interfering with the client's willingness to participate in the chain right now. "Given all these important reasons to do a chain analysis on important behaviors, what's getting in the way for you right now?" It is important here to focus only on this moment and not get caught up in all the reasons the client has ever historically not wanted to do chains. While a discussion regarding all the reasons might make sense at some point in the future, in this instance it would largely serve as a distraction from the chain, thereby reinforcing avoidance behavior.

The therapist can also take an alternate approach by using highlighting and/or hypothesis generation to label an interference. This refers to naming what is getting in the way, which can also function as validation by helping the client feel understood by the therapist. Some examples of what this might look like are "Here's our friend shame again, showing up and getting in the way of us figuring this out!"; "I'm thinking you might be feeling hopeless right now and that's interfering with you wanting to jump in and do this with me"; "This shutting down of yours feels similar to what happened a few weeks ago and you later told me that you weren't sure that you wanted to stop your drinking after all. Is that going through your mind again right now?" These examples show ways to zero-in on obstacles that are interfering with the chain and also to acknowledge them as obstacles, rather than unique, independent problems. For example, a client might say "I just don't feel like doing it today," without recognizing that this "not feeling like it" is a common problem for her that shows up across multiple situations and contexts. By highlighting the problem as a core one (see Rizvi & Sayrs, 2018), the therapist can work to motivate the client to push through and address it: "If we can get you to jump into doing the chain analysis with me right now, we can figure out every other problem in your life." The therapist is highlighting the value of the chain that extends far past this one particular instance. It also can serve a motivator for pushing through with a difficult task. Table 2.2 summarizes the above strategies.

When Deficits in Episodic Memory Cause Avoidance

Some clients may avoid chains due to skills deficits in remembering and processing information in a sequential fashion. Lynch, Chapman, Rosenthal, Kuo, and Linehan (2006) wrote about how the process of chain analyses might be an important agent of change in DBT because it may improve the episodic aspect of autobiographical memory. Deficits in episodic memory mean that a person might not be able to remember important aspects of an event including specifics related to what happened, when it happened, and where it happened. While there are many instances in which problems with this kind of memory might not be so important (e.g., try to recall your dinner from last Wednesday night), one can imagine that episodic memory as it relates to significant events

TABLE 2.2. Strategies for Countering Chain Analysis Avoidance Later in Treatment

- Ask the client to generate the reasons for chain analyses.
- Briefly assess what is interfering with the client's willingness to do a chain analysis right now or test hypotheses about the obstacle.
- Use the assessment information to elicit the client's commitment to move forward with the chain analysis.
- Remain a constant supporter of the use of chain analysis.

is quite important when it comes to learning how events in a sequence are tied together. For example, a client saying, "I can't really remember what happened, it just seemed that all of a sudden a crack pipe was in my hand and I was lighting up" is indicative of such a problem. If clients have such deficits throughout their lives, one can easily see how it would be difficult to determine how to reduce the risk of using drugs in the future since the key contributors are unknown. Thus, the review of the relationships among thoughts, emotions, and behaviors with the therapist via the chain analysis may help the client improve his or her abilities to see patterns. Further, improving episodic memory may lead to improved problem solving for future situations (Williams, Conway, & Cohen, 2008). How does that process work? Repeated in-session chain analyses can help clients more clearly recognize problematic patterns of behavior as they take place in their lives. Improved awareness of these patterns and sequences of events can lead the client to remember how similar situations in the past have led to ineffective behaviors with negative consequences. These memories will increase the likelihood that a client will change course in the sequence of events so that more functional outcomes can occur.

Problems with episodic memory among our clients were clearly brought to life for me early in my career as a DBT trainer when I had the opportunity to co-lead a training with the fabulous teacher Dr. Elizabeth Simpson of Harvard Medical School. Liz told a story about an interaction with a client that clearly demonstrated the deficits that some of our clients have regarding episodic memory. Liz tells the story this way:

> "It was the early days in DBT with a young woman who chronically self-injured by swallowing pens and cutting herself. I was attempting a chain analysis of a cutting incident with her and it kept getting derailed. That is, we would put one or two steps together (. . . so I went to the house manager and asked her for a pen, and she said, 'No, not right now') and I would say something like 'Did that hurt your feelings?' and she would suddenly say, 'So I was talking to the nurse.' What nurse? When? 'On Tuesday.' But we were talking about Thursday . . . and so on. There was a lot of disjunctions and confusion. And I started to notice that I was getting extremely frustrated. In one of my less stellar moments as a therapist, I said, 'Let's start with today. You were waiting downstairs in the waiting area. I came down and got you. We walked upstairs.' Something about the pitch and tone of my voice was alarming and she drew back and looked at

me with great big eyes. In a moment of dysregulation, I said loudly and in exasperation, 'Have you not noticed that life moves inevitably moment by moment in one direction from left to right?' There was a long pause and then she silently shook her head no. And the penny dropped. She couldn't sequence events in time. And it just blew my mind to realize how difficult life would be if events seem to arise in a disconnected way."

I appreciate this story for many reasons, not least of which is the fact that sometimes when we feel least effective as a therapist, we discover something that radically shifts the treatment. I think this story clearly demonstrates the problems many of our clients have and why doing a chain analysis is both so difficult and so important. The capacity to understand how a behavior occurs *in context* is a necessary prerequisite to learning how to change it. If you are unaware of the dozens of "warning signs" that indicate that a target behavior is very likely to occur, then you are unable to effectively strategize about how to change behavior.

Of course, not all clients have deficits in this area as severe as Liz's client did. Doing the first few chain analyses with a new client will help the therapist assess the degree to which memory impairments occur. Although there might be urges to avoid doing chains with someone with memory problems (e.g., "She's not able to do it" or "She needs more time in treatment before we start doing chains"), I would argue that jumping in anyway will serve a couple of functions. In fact, I suggest that the greater the magnitude of the memory problems, the *more* critical it is to do chain analyses. One reason is that it will communicate to the client (and you!) that chains are a vital part of treatment regardless of the obstacles. Two, the process of repeatedly doing chains will ultimately help identify and address some of the memory problems. For example, a client who says that "I just found a knife in my hand; I have no idea how it got there," will benefit from attention paid to zeroing-in on the moments that preceded this instant and slowly learning how to put the pieces together.

If memory impairment is one of the obstacles to doing chains, a therapist will want to rely heavily on orientation in order to try to get the client on board. For example:

"I know that it's very difficult for you to analyze behavior in this really fine-tuned way. In the past, when we have attempted to do it, you have said that you don't remember large chunks of time and/or you don't remember the order in which events occurred over time. These problems with memory are pretty common and likely are one of the reasons why it's been so difficult for you to change your behavior over time! That is why I think it is so important that we slow down and really look at this self-harm event from this past week. It's OK if you don't remember all the pieces right now. My hope is that the more we do these analyses, the more we'll be able to fill in the gaps. That will help us figure out the best way to solve these problems together! Sound good?"

As with previous examples, there is a heavy dose of validation here that involves normalizing and expressing understanding of the problem. This validation improves the likelihood that orientation will be effective because it highlights the unique factors of the person. As a corollary, imagine hearing someone say to you, "We are going to work on getting you to eat healthy because it's good for all people to eat in a more healthful way." While this may represent a fundamental fact about what contributes to longevity and healthy living, it likely does not evoke in you a strong desire to start eating more vegetables. Now consider this version: "I know that there are many obstacles that get in the way of you eating in a healthy way. This is true for a lot of people but may be especially true for you given the circumstances of your busy life. That said, I think it's really important for you to work on this with me because eating in a more healthful manner will ultimately lead you to reach many of your desired goals." Although still somewhat vague, it is a far more personal entreaty to get you to work on changing your behavior using validation and identification of potential obstacles. It also highlights the importance of linking to a client's goals in the orientation. If I was trying to "sell" you on a healthy diet, I would likely have far more success in doing so with the second version. When it comes to orientation, we want to increase the likelihood that a client is on board with our tasks in treatment. Thus, the importance of "selling" it to the client in a meaningful and personal way cannot be overstated.

How to Increase Collaboration in Chain Analyses

There are no set, explicit rules about how to do a chain analysis. Ultimately, what should govern how therapists conduct them is their effectiveness. To make them effective, it is extremely important to keep the process of chains as collaborative as possible. The chain is not meant to exist only within the mind of the therapist. Many clients early in treatment exhibit a passive problem-solving style in which they expect other people to solve their problems for them. Thus, increasing collaboration also likely improves the client's skills with active problem solving and being an agent of change, rather than a passive recipient of others' actions. Thus, a therapist might say something like the following as part of the orientation to the process of the chain:

> "It's really important to me that this task be something that we do together. In order for this treatment to work, I want to help you to become your own DBT therapist over time. That means working together on these chains and me telling you the reasons why I'm asking what I'm asking along the way."

While keeping in mind the function of the chain analysis, I provide here some tips that might help your overall effectiveness in conducting them and having them lead more effectively to change. It is important to note that orientation will likely be necessary for each of these guidelines as well, so I provide an example for each as to how this orientation might be provided.

Make the Process Visual and Tangible

I strongly encourage the use of a whiteboard, blackboard, or writing pad to map out the chain with the client. Many therapists find that working with the chain in a visual manner helps keep them on task and organized. Many clients also report finding it helpful to see it all visually laid out and they begin to see how various parts of the sequence are connected and intertwined. You should be careful not to assume that just because it's clear to you, it's also clear to the client. Having a point of visual reference that both the therapist and the client look at together also decreases the likelihood of miscommunication or misunderstanding. A client could say, after looking at the chain on the board, "No, actually my feelings of anger didn't show up there [pointing to link]. It showed up a few minutes later [pointing to another link]." This sort of information would be difficult to obtain if the therapist was keeping the entire chain in her head. As described above, many times, our clients lack the awareness of the sequence of events—that's why they are in therapy to begin with. Even if you do a chain analysis on your own behavior, it may only become clear when you see it visually.

> "I have found it really helpful to use this whiteboard here to write out the chain as we do it. There's many reasons for this: it helps keep us both on track, it helps in a visual way to show how everything that happened that night was connected, it helps make sure we both see things the same way, and it often really makes clear where the possible points of intervention could be for the future."

Similarly, find a way to give the client a copy of the chain analysis at the end of the session. The copy can then be reviewed by the client during the week. Most of the clients in my program take a photo of the completed chain with their cell phones. Some colleagues of mine recommend using carbon paper to write out the chain in session and then the therapist and client can each take a copy.

> "Now that we've finished this first pass of this chain, I want you take a picture of it with your phone and look at it during the week. In particular, I want you to see if there was anything important that we may have missed as you think about it more."

Audio-Record the Chain Analysis

An often overlooked strategy in DBT is to have clients audio-record the session and listen to it during the week as homework (Linehan, 1993). There are many functions of this task (see Rizvi & Roman, 2019); one of them is to enhance the client's memory for the session and the information that was generated during it. This might be especially important if the client is dysregulated, or experiences intense emotions during the conduct of the chain analysis. Although orientation to audio recording in general will be delivered somewhat differently, an example of how it might be used specifically for chain analyses follows:

> "When you listen to the recording of this session this week, I'd like you to pay special attention to the part where we did the chain analysis because I noticed that some of those questions were difficult for you to answer and you were experiencing some pretty intense emotions. I don't want you to forget some of the really important

work we did in analyzing this behavior today. So listen carefully to the chain analysis section of the session, write down your thoughts or anything else you remember about the sequence, and let me know next week if you have any questions about it."

If audio-recording of the entire sessions is not being done on a weekly basis for whatever reason, a therapist can ask the client to turn on his or her voice recorder just for the chain portion of the session.

Involve the Client

The strategies listed thus far are all aimed at increasing collaboration. However, even with the implementation of these approaches, a therapist might still find the client difficult to engage or only half-heartedly going through the motions of the chain. Thus, it is important to look for any opportunity to increase the involvement of the client. Some of this can be done by returning to the rationale, linking it to client goals, and generating hope, but all of these are verbal techniques which may not help when the client is shutting down. If a therapist notices a client begin to shut down or tune out during a chain analysis, it could be a perfect opportunity to try to activate the client in a more physical way in order to increase engagement. Fluctuating stylistic strategies (discussed in Chapter 4) can help to engage the client mentally by capturing his or her attention.

Observing videos of therapists conducting chains over the year, I have often noticed that in order to write out the chain on a whiteboard, the therapist has to turn his or her back toward the client. Watching the client in those moments, I frequently observe them looking away, looking down, or otherwise looking unengaged with what the therapist is writing. In many circumstances, this takes away from the whole point of writing the chain out on the board! In such circumstances, I recommend that the therapist ask the client to get up and take over by writing the chain on the whiteboard him- or herself instead of the therapist doing all the work. Sometimes just asking a client to stand up, stand near the whiteboard, and continue engaging with the process of the chain can be useful, as it provides an uptick in energy.

"I appreciate you doing the chain with me and I also know that it can be difficult to sustain attention, especially when it takes me a while to write things out. How about we take turns? I write some things out as we discuss them and then I pass the marker to you to take over? What do you think?"

If a whiteboard is not being used, having the client write out the chain on paper will also serve to increase his or her involvement in the process.

Assign a Chain Analysis as Homework

Once you have conducted a couple of analyses in session, you can consider assigning the client a homework assignment of completing a chain analyses him- or herself following a behavior of clinical interest. This assignment can serve a couple of functions: one, if the client completes the analysis shortly after the event occurs, there is a lowered chance that faded memory interferes with the process. Two, this assignment has the client practice the skill of doing a chain analysis him- or herself and attempt to determine the important variables. This assignment would then need to be carefully reviewed in the next session. There are handouts and worksheets related to chain analysis in the second edition of the skills manual (Linehan, 2015); these can be used for the assignment.

> "I've noticed that we have done a few chain analyses in sessions and yet the behavior continues to occur despite our best attempts at coming up with solutions. I'm wondering if too much time is going by between when the behavior happens and when we analyze it, which might mean we are not getting all the information we need. Now that you know how to do a chain, I'd like you to start writing out a chain as soon as possible after the behavior occurs."

Remind Yourself about the Importance of Chain Analysis

A final guideline for increasing collaboration for chains in therapy is to continue to remind yourself of the importance of the chain analysis and the information it yields. This reminder is important and meant to be an antidote to the sometimes negative feedback we can get from clients who want to avoid the nuanced dissection of their behaviors. I have often seen therapists slowly ask fewer and fewer questions when they are working with clients who are resistant to doing chains or who display all sorts of aversive behaviors when a therapist attempts to home in on a target behavior. Therapists can get shaped by this behavior, and not even realize that they are colluding in the avoidance behavior.

Of course, this means that you actually believe chains are an important aspect of the treatment! If you find yourself on the fence, I hope that this book really makes the case for why chain analyses are vital to thorough assessment of target behaviors and subsequent solutions for those behaviors. I also hope that you conduct chain analyses on yourself and your own target behaviors. Doing so will help you get more practice with the process as well as become more aware of obstacles that come up for you that might help you understand similar obstacles with your clients. It then can be very effective to use self-disclosure with your clients around the process of chains.

> "You just said that this process seems tedious to you and I can understand that because you've never been asked to look at a behavior this closely before. However, I can tell you from personal experience that chains are very useful at helping us ultimately change in the ways that we want and feel like we have more control over our own behaviors. I used chains to cure myself of a snoozing behavior problem I used to have. It wasn't until I did repeated chains on my snoozing that I recognized all the different things I could try to reduce it. Before I did chains, I just tried the willpower model, which just doesn't work that well. I imagine it doesn't work that well for you either. So let's do this!"

In this chapter, I provided a rationale for the importance of orienting clients to the task of chain analysis, ways in which the orientation can be provided, how to use orientation when a client is willing and when a client is not willing, and general methods to increase collaboration in the process of the chain. Thus, this chapter focused on increasing collaboration with the procedure by "selling" the chain analysis as a process that is important and worth doing. Now that the basic elements of the chain have been described and the ways in which you can get started doing chains in treatment have been outlined, it is time to move into the more nuts and bolts of chains in treatment. Since the functions of chains often change over time, I turn first to using chain analyses to "get to know a behavior."

CHAPTER 3

Getting to Know the Target Behavior
ASSESSING A PROBLEM THE FIRST TIME

I n this chapter, I focus specifically on the experience of doing chain analyses in order to learn about the target behavior and identify the various components of the chain for the first time. These chain analyses can occur as early as the first or second session when therapists are starting to assess a behavior that they don't know anything about. Such chains also occur throughout treatment, for example, when a new target behavior shows up that has to be addressed or when the client has made significant strides on addressing his or her primary problem behavior and now therapy is turning to the next target of treatment. There are aspects to these early chains that make them quite different from chains that might be done the third or fourth (or 138th!) time a behavior occurs.

Since the first chain ever conducted is often the clients' first exposure to the process of such in-depth behavioral analysis, these early chains "set the stage" for treatment in many ways: they highlight the fundamental behavioral approach that informs the treatment, they gather important information about the target(s) of treatment that will lead to subsequent solution generation and implementation, and they help to inform case conceptualization and treatment planning. Using the principles designed to increase collaboration highlighted in the previous chapter, the therapist also communicates the importance and value of this task starting with the very first chain.

For the clinician, it is important to remember to adopt a "beginner's mind" for the assessment and not add assumptions or jump steps because you think you know how pieces are related. By making assumptions, you run the risk of missing important idiographic details that may be critical for the analysis. Given that this is often the first time a client is speaking about a serious problem in such specific detail, you can expect that there might be client shame, embarrassment, and/or urges to conceal. If a client conceals an important aspect of the chain the first time, it becomes harder and harder for him or her to reveal it later on, in part because he or she then also has to admit to lying behavior. Thus, I have found that incorporating a nonjudgmental, matter-of-fact style to the beginner's mind stance is crucial for creating a context in which the client is most likely to reveal all. That said, it is of course quite possible that not all is revealed in these early chains for myriad reasons. (These reasons, and solutions to this problem, are addressed in Chapter 6.) Finally, keep in mind that these early chains are often works in progress. It is important to recognize that the first occurrence of a careful analysis of a behavior takes time. Therapists often feel rushed to complete a "perfect" chain in a short amount of time. Although I will be providing suggestions for how to learn to zero-in on critical points later, and thus reduce the overall amount of time spent on the chains, I am reminded here of a favorite quote of mine. Listening to a radio interview with a famous actor, she recounted that a director once said to her, "We don't have a lot of time, so we have to work very slowly." This paradoxical comment so embodies the nature of assessment in DBT that I use it frequently with trainees as well as clients.

- Adopt a beginner's mind.
- Be nonjudgmental and matter-of-fact.
- Don't rush.

In this chapter, I will use three case examples—Sasha, Laurie, and Isaac—to show some ways in which these early chains might be conducted. Specifically, I highlight: how to identify the target behavior of the chain analysis (the "problem behavior" component), how to assess the behavior and the five components of the chain in a way that orients the client to the procedure, including why such an in-depth analysis is critical for increasing the effectiveness of the treatment. These are relatively simple examples that don't have the myriad of choice points that often arise in more complex clinical situations.

Chain Analysis of Sasha's Drinking Behavior

Sasha enters into treatment for help with depression. She does not engage in any life-threatening behavior like suicide attempts or self-injury and denies thinking about suicide, but the therapist discovers in the initial intake session that Sasha drinks copious amounts of alcohol, up to a pint of vodka several times a week. Even though Sasha believes that the alcohol helps her deal with her depression, the therapist describes for her all the ways in which alcohol is known to exacerbate depression and suggests that, in fact, her depression likely won't improve unless she first stops drinking. Given this information, and working together, they agree to make drinking the highest target for the initial stage of treatment. After assessing other relevant history and current functioning in the first two sessions, the therapist adds chain analysis of a drinking episode to his agenda for the third session. He orients Sasha to the content and process of the chain and proceeds with her consent. In the transcript below of the chain between Sasha and the therapist, I highlight the components of the chain that the therapist is assessing as well as the incorporation of other principles previously discussed.

Defining the Target Behavior and Prompting Event

THERAPIST: Given that drinking occurs several times a week, it might be difficult to focus on one particular episode without thinking of all the similarities or differences with other nights. However, I still think it would be most helpful for us to start with one particular night so that I can get to understand what happens for you. Looking back over the past few days, were there any nights that stand out to you as being particularly difficult?

SASHA: Not really. They are all a blur.

THERAPIST: OK. Given that, how about we focus on last night since that might be easiest for you to remember. I'm going to write this out on the whiteboard here as we go along. Did you drink last night?

SASHA: Yes.

THERAPIST: How much did you drink? [beginning the chain by focusing on the target behavior]

SASHA: Don't know exactly but probably about eight shots worth.

THERAPIST: What time was this? [target behavior]

SASHA: I started after my boyfriend left, probably around 10:00.

THERAPIST: And the drinking lasted for how long? [target behavior]

SASHA: I was watching TV and drinking at the same time. I think I passed out on the couch before the show even ended so probably less than an hour.

THERAPIST: OK, so you drank about eight shots of vodka between 10:00 and 11:00. Is this a typical pattern for you? [Although he is focusing on one specific episode, since this is the first chain of a treatment target, it is helpful to know how similar this is to other experiences. If this was extremely *dis*similar, it might not be as useful a chain for an initial assessment.]

SASHA: Yeah, this is usually what happens. I fall asleep and then wake up a few hours later feeling like crap.

THERAPIST: OK, we'll get to that in a minute. Let's go back to last night's drinking. How did you drink? Did you pour yourself shots or mix it with something or drink out of the bottle or what? [target behavior— really trying to "see" it in his mind's eye]

SASHA: I usually drink more than I set out to. I start by pouring myself shots and then just start swigging out of the bottle.

THERAPIST: So last night, how many shots did you pour before you started drinking from the bottle? [anchoring to last night]

SASHA: I think three. I can't remember exactly.

THERAPIST: This is helpful. You're doing great. After three shots, you started drinking from the bottle and think you had a few more shots-worth before you passed out? All while you were watching a TV show?

SASHA: Yes, sounds about right.

THERAPIST: OK, so going back in time a bit. When did you first start having urges to drink last night or realizing that you were going to drink? [assessing prompting event]

SASHA: I don't know if I had a specific realization about it. But I do remember thinking when Brian [boyfriend] was over that I couldn't wait for him to leave so I could start drinking. He doesn't like it when I drink because he says it makes me "sloppy."

THERAPIST: So you had the thought "I wish he would leave so I can start drinking"?

SASHA: Yup.

THERAPIST: What time was this?

SASHA: Just as we were finishing dinner, around 9:00, I think. We were sitting in front of the TV together and I wanted to drink so I started reminding him that he had to get up early today for work. I was hoping that he would take the hint and leave.

THERAPIST: Do you remember if anything in particular set off these thoughts for you about wanting to drink and wanting him to leave?

SASHA: Nothing I can think of. Maybe it was just the time of night. I was feeling low, just wanting to drink and sleep.

THERAPIST: OK, feeling low or depressed might have been a vulnerability for you—we'll come back to that. But I'm wondering if something set these thoughts off. Even if it feels to you right now that they come in out of the blue, usually it's possible to find some sort of cue or "trigger" for such thoughts. [orienting to idea of "prompting event"] What was happening with you or with you and Brian right before you started having thoughts about drinking, do you remember?

SASHA: I don't remember!

THERAPIST: That makes sense, I'm sure it all seems like a blur right now. If you were to put yourself back in that situation this moment—sitting on the couch with Brian around 9:00 P.M., watching TV—what goes through your mind?

SASHA: I'm tired. I didn't sleep well the night before. I want to go to sleep. I know I'm not going to go to sleep unless I have something to drink; otherwise my racing thoughts will keep me up. I gotta get them to stop so I can have some peace.

THERAPIST: Great job with identifying those thoughts! Even if they aren't exactly the same as what happened last night, it sounds pretty believable to me that you would be having thoughts like those. Does it seem that way to you?

SASHA: Yeah, those are pretty common thoughts.

THERAPIST: So, for the moment, we're going to label these thoughts about wanting to go to sleep and thinking alcohol will help with that as the prompting event. I don't know you well enough yet to know if there are other events that set off this type of thinking or not but I think this gives us a good starting point.

So far, the therapist has identified and clearly described the problem behavior. He has also identified the prompting event for the chain. Notice that this is not an example where there is a very clear prompting event that controls the subsequent chain of events. An example of a clearer prompting event would be if Sasha said she wasn't thinking about drinking at all until she and her boyfriend had a fight about dinner and then that led to her drinking. In that case, we would identify "fight with boyfriend" as the prompting event. However, with more frequently occurring behavior, it is often the case that the prompting event is less concrete. What's important here is that the therapist not get bogged down with trying to find *the* prompting event and instead be flexible in determining the appropriate starting point that is proximal to the problem behavior (see discussion in Chapter 1).

> Don't get bogged down trying to find *the* prompting event. Be flexible in determining the point proximal to the problem behavior.

Identifying Links

What would follow next in this chain is the therapist asking Sasha to fill in the steps between thoughts about wanting to go to sleep and drinking the first shot. According to her report, this would be about 1 hour in duration. Let's imagine that, with the therapist's help, Sasha identifies the following links:

1. Thought that in order to get to bed quickly, Brian would have to leave soon. [cognition]
2. Said to Brian, "Don't you have to get up early tomorrow for your job?" [behavior]
3. Brian said something like "Yeah, but I don't feel like getting up."
4. Noticed irritation and disgust. [emotions]
5. Started noisily cleaning up dishes in the kitchen [behavior] and thinking about how he should leave. [cognitions]
6. Anger increases.

7. Starts a fight with boyfriend by calling him lazy and telling him he can't lose another job. [behavior]

8. Fight occurs for about 20 minutes during which they just "hash out all the things we hate about each other." [behavior]

9. Intense anger, shame, and sadness.

10. Brian says, "Forget it, I can't take this anymore tonight" and leaves.

11. Notices relief and thought "Thank God he's gone." [emotion and cognition]

12. Gets vodka bottle and shot glass from bedroom closet where she stores it. [behavior]

13. Settles into couch and pours first shot. [behavior]

14. Notices relief and some excitement. [emotion]

15. Starts drinking. [problem behavior]

There are a few things to note about these links, and the process of obtaining them. As described in Chapter 1, the primary aim of evaluating the connection between each link is to be able to understand how the person got from Point A (the prompting event) to Point B (the target behavior). The first time a chain is conducted on a specific behavior, the therapist often does not have a clear sense yet of what the controlling variables might be, because this is the first time he or she is hearing about how the events unfold. Thus, the first chain of a problem behavior might look very different than a chain on the same problem behavior conducted later in treatment. In early sessions, when the therapist is trying to get to know the client, the focus is most often on broad strokes. For example, in this third session with Sasha, the therapist has identified important variables to be addressed in treatment: irritability, "picking a fight," and the relief from negative emotions achieved through her anticipation of drinking. This level of information could be enough knowledge at this point in treatment. In subsequent sessions, especially if the drinking behavior is not changing, the therapist might home in on any one of these areas and get much more detail in order to understand its relevance for the subsequent drinking (see Chapter 6).

Notice also that some of these links raise questions about Sasha that may be important to further assess outside the context of the chain.

For example, it might be important to know what her boyfriend knows about her drinking, what he communicates to her about her drinking, the nature of their relationship and fights in general, and so forth. These can inform the therapist about Sasha's life more generally as well as possible broader solutions to suggest that operate outside the context of this chain (e.g., reducing relationship conflict more generally would likely lead to fewer problem behaviors, including drinking). The therapist may ask some of these questions in the first chain but it is very important that he or she not lose sight of the chain. In other words, he or she can take a couple of detours to check out the scenery but should always come back to the main road in the service of getting to the destination. Otherwise, he or she runs the risk of losing sight of the end goal: finding effective solutions that will have an impact on the target behavior in the future. A novice therapist might want to avoid taking these detours in the first few sessions until he or she has mastered the process of chain analyses. Once the process becomes more familiar, the therapist can practice going back and forth between the detours and the primary route.

Identifying Consequences

Returning to Sasha's chain of drinking behavior, we now have information on the prompting event, links, and problem behavior. Another domain to assess is consequences. Remember that short-term consequences are often more critical in controlling the behavior than those longer-term consequences (see Chapter 1). The conversation might go like this:

THERAPIST: What happened when you started drinking?

SASHA: I just kept drinking until I passed out, like I said.

THERAPIST: No. Let me be more specific—what did you notice immediately after you had the first shot? [anchoring to immediate consequences]

SASHA: Oh. I think I remember liking the taste. Well, not liking the taste exactly, but liking the sensation. And then sort of feeling like "Finally! I get to zone out."

THERAPIST: Was that a relief feeling? Or excitement? [focusing on labeling emotions]

SASHA: Maybe a little bit of both.

THERAPIST: OK, so the immediate consequences to drinking seem pretty positive. What happened as you continued drinking?

SASHA: I sort of just went into automatic pilot. Kept drinking and started swigging from the bottle. After a while, I don't remember very much and then I woke up on the couch a few hours later.

THERAPIST: When you were continuing to drink, did you still feel relief and excitement or did the feelings change? [focusing on emotions]

SASHA: I think I just became numb.

THERAPIST: Is that a positive feeling for you? [assessment without assumption]

SASHA: Better than feeling depressed, yeah.

THERAPIST: OK, that's important for us to know. And then what were the longer-term consequences of last night's drinking, if any? What happened when you woke up?

SASHA: I feel awful. My head hurts and is foggy, I feel nauseous. I go to my bed and try to sleep more but it's usually tossing and turning for a few hours.

THERAPIST: And is that what happened this morning as well? [remaining focused on single event]

SASHA: Yeah, until I had to get up to come here.

The therapist has now acquired knowledge about the potential consequences— both positive and negative—for the client. As I have mentioned before, the therapist and the client could engage in a wide-ranging discussion about how drinking affects her in broader ways such as effects of drinking on social and occupational functioning. The therapist would likely want to return to these topics at another point, especially if he or she needs to work on her commitment to stop drinking by developing a pros and cons list or by emphasizing the negative consequences of drinking.

Vulnerability Factors

At this point in the assessment, the therapist has adequately addressed the sequence from the prompting event through to consequences. What remains to be uncovered are vulnerability factors. Here's what that assessment might look like.

THERAPIST: Let's go back, for a moment, to the beginning of the chain. You mentioned earlier that you were feeling low, or depressed. But I know you've said that feeling down is pretty standard for you these days. Was there anything that stood out to you about last night in particular that may have made you more vulnerable to those thoughts about wanting to go to sleep?

SASHA: Well, I was feeling depressed and really tired.

THERAPIST: And that sounds painful. Were those feelings stronger than usual last night? Or do you feel that way every night?

SASHA: I feel that way almost every night.

THERAPIST: And yet, you don't drink every night. Anything different about last night? In other words, was there anything last night that made you more vulnerable than other nights when you don't end up drinking?

SASHA: Hmm. I'm not sure. Nothing that I can remember.

THERAPIST: OK, we'll keep an eye out for that in the future. My guess is that there are days when there are things that happen that make you more vulnerable to drinking than other days. We just might not know what those things are yet. We'll figure it out.

SASHA: OK.

In this example, clearly identified vulnerability factors appear to be lacking. It's important to remember that, especially in early chains, a therapist may take what he or she can get and note that more information will be revealed as he or she gets to know the client and the different situations that prompt the same problem behavior. A novice therapist might be inclined to stick to this point and insist upon finding a vulnerability factor before moving on. Or a therapist may look to more enduring features (e.g., "alcohol dependence" or "depression") as a vulnerability factor. However, as Sasha's therapist points out here, Sasha almost always feels depressed, as per her report, so that wouldn't explain why she was more vulnerable to drinking *on that day*. However, it could be that Sasha's depression feels worse on particular days, and on those days she is more vulnerable to drinking (and conversely, she doesn't drink on days when her depression is milder). However, Sasha is not yet aware of this potential pattern. Using a diary card to track emotion states and problem behaviors is one tool that helps to elucidate the relationship between key variables over time.

Look for why the client was more vulnerable to the problem behavior *on that day*. If this isn't clear, don't insist on finding vulnerability factors before moving on.

At this point, the therapist would consider the chain analysis of Sasha's drinking behavior last night to be complete, or detailed "enough," to proceed to solution analysis, discussed in Chapter 5. The visual of the chain on the whiteboard would look something like Figure 3.1.

This analysis fulfilled the goals of a chain in early treatment: it allowed the therapist to get to know more about Sasha and her identified top target of treatment; it began to identify possible controlling variables, and it indicated potential points of intervention. As suggested in the beginning of this chapter, a chain analysis very early in treatment is helpful for a number of reasons, which were exemplified by showing how the chain analysis was conducted on Sasha's drinking behavior. One is that the therapist starts to learn more about the client and obtains information about the client's life that will be helpful for the rest of therapy. For example, in this brief chain, the therapist now knows more about the typical pattern of her drinking, her problems with sleep and interpersonal effectiveness, and her mood states. In addition, the variables that show up in this early chain might be the same links that show up in chains of all future treatment targets. While these factors are as yet unknown, the process of looking for parallels starts with the early chains. By drawing parallels, therapists can identify core problems that are most in need of intervention (Rizvi & Sayrs, 2018).

Chain Analysis of Laurie's Self-Injurious Behavior

When conducting chain analyses with more high-risk behaviors, such as suicidal behavior and nonsuicidal self-injury, it may be tempting to stray from the structure of the chain to solve the problem more quickly. However, with such behaviors there is even more need for careful and precise assessment so that an *effective* solution, not just any solution, is likely to be identified. Thus, suicidal behavior and nonsuicidal self-injury (NSSI) are addressed just like any other behavior. In the following example, an episode of self-harm is analyzed in which there is a longer length of time between the prompting event and the problem behavior. Strategies for how to focus on the key links (rather than every single second) are highlighted.

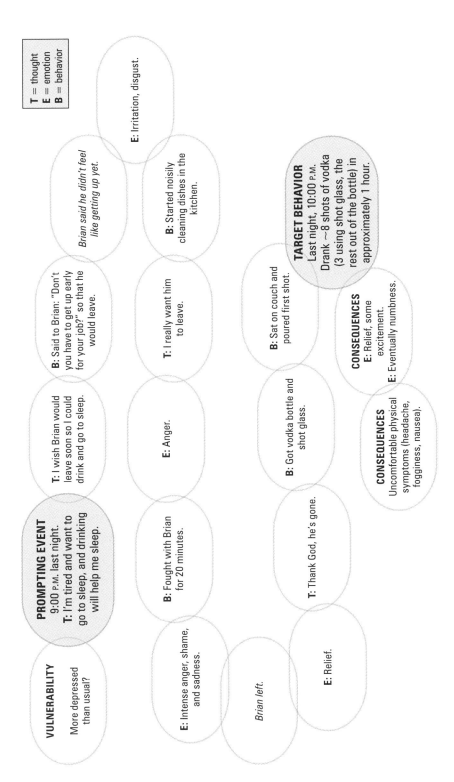

FIGURE 3.1. Chain analysis of Sasha's drinking behavior.

T = thought
E = emotion
B = behavior

VULNERABILITY

More depressed than usual?

PROMPTING EVENT

9:00 P.M. last night.
T: I'm tired and want to go to sleep, and drinking will help me sleep.

T: I wish Brian would leave soon so I could drink and go to sleep.

B: Said to Brian: "Don't you have to get up early for your job?" so that he would leave.

Brian said he didn't feel like getting up yet.

E: Irritation, disgust.

B: Started noisily cleaning dishes in the kitchen.

T: I really want him to leave.

E: Anger.

B: Fought with Brian for 20 minutes.

E: Intense anger, shame, and sadness.

Brian left.

T: Thank God, he's gone.

E: Relief.

B: Got vodka bottle and shot glass.

B: Sat on couch and poured first shot.

TARGET BEHAVIOR

Last night, 10:00 P.M.
Drank ~8 shots of vodka (3 using shot glass, the rest out of the bottle) in approximately 1 hour.

CONSEQUENCES

E: Relief, some excitement.
E: Eventually numbness.

CONSEQUENCES

Uncomfortable physical symptoms (headache, fogginess, nausea).

53

Laurie, a 28-year-old woman, presented to treatment with suicide ideation and self-harm behavior in the form of cutting on her legs with razor blades. The first few sessions had been spent carefully assessing and managing suicide risk, as well as completing other tasks associated with the first few sessions of DBT. Despite Laurie's commitment in Session 1 not to kill or harm herself, she continued to cut once or twice a week for the first 4 weeks of treatment. Given other tasks for therapy, the therapist had not yet conducted a detailed chain analysis; however, she did get Laurie to commit to removing all razor blades from her apartment and not buying new ones. In Session 5, the therapist turns her attention explicitly to assessing self-injury. At this point, the therapist is still getting to know Laurie and the controlling variables of her cutting behavior.

Defining the Target Behavior

THERAPIST: Laurie, we have got to figure out what is happening with your cutting so that we can get you to stop doing it. Are you willing to do a chain analysis with me?

LAURIE: I guess so. I'm just not sure how we're ever going to get it to stop. I've been doing it for most of my life by now. [Laurie was 13 when she first cut herself.]

THERAPIST: It's true, it's been a long time for you and therefore it's a behavior that is really strong right now. Our task is to figure out all the critical variables that are related to cutting, and find new behaviors that are more healthy and effective and then practice those new behaviors over and over again until they become even more strong. Are you with me?

LAURIE: Yes, that sounds good.

THERAPIST: OK, let's choose one of the two instances of cutting to focus on for the chain. Do you have a preference?

LAURIE: It might make sense to talk about yesterday since I remember that one better.

THERAPIST: Great idea, let's do it. [*Stands up and starts to work on whiteboard in full view of Laurie*]. So, typically the problem behavior is cutting on your legs with a razor blade. Is that what happened yesterday? [target behavior definition]

LAURIE: Yup.

THERAPIST: Can you describe it for me in a bit more detail? Where did you cut exactly? How long and deep was the cut?

LAURIE: I cut here on my upper thigh so that no one can see the scar. I made about three cuts, each about an inch long. It drew blood but not a lot. Since I got rid of my razors after the last session, I used some scissors that I had lying around.

THERAPIST: OK, I'm very glad to hear that you followed through on getting rid of your razors and of course much less glad to hear that you used something else. But we'll get to that. So the problem behavior is cutting three times on your upper leg with scissors. What time was this?

LAURIE: About 10:00 last night.

At this point, the therapist has defined the problem behavior in specific terms. She is focusing on a specific instance, rather than speaking in generalities. The behavior is also anchored in time and a new method (scissors) has been identified, indicating that a solution that was implemented last week (getting rid of the preferred method) was not totally successful at eliminating the problem behavior.

Identifying the Prompting Event

THERAPIST: Let's move backward in a time a bit. When did you first think about cutting?

LAURIE: Honestly, I had it in the back of my mind as an option all day. I sort of woke up thinking about it.

THERAPIST: Hmm, is that typical for you or was there something different about yesterday?

LAURIE: That's sort of typical. Since we've been talking about it so much in sessions and working on stopping it, it's almost like I'm thinking about it more.

THERAPIST: Definitely not what we want of course! That said, something that will be important for us to figure out is how you can have thoughts about cutting without actually cutting. So if the urges were sort of in the background for you most of yesterday, what do you think was the event that set you down the path toward cutting? [Attempting to identify the prompting event. Sometimes this can be done by asking when urges to engage in the behavior started and then identifying the event that immediately preceded that urge. However, it many cases, like this one, the client either cannot identify a specific time point at which urges occurred *or* he or she reports that the urges are a near constant presence. Mindfulness skills will help with this later.]

LAURIE: I came home from work and started to think about how I have no friends, nothing to do that feels important to me, and I started getting increasingly anxious that nothing in my life is ever going to change.

THERAPIST: So hopelessness and anxiety showed up?

LAURIE: Yes, it feels so terrible and overwhelming and nothing I do seems to make it go away.

THERAPIST: OK, we're going to have to work on that for sure. In terms of last night, what time did you get home from work?

LAURIE: Around 6:00, I think.

THERAPIST: OK, so let's focus on that as the prompting event for the sake of the chain. Would you say that urges to cut intensified after you got home and felt anxious or did that happen before you got home from work?

LAURIE: It didn't really start to feel intense until after I got home. There were times at work during the day when I wasn't thinking about it as much.

Vulnerability Factors

THERAPIST: Good to know. OK, so the prompting event was arriving home around 6:00 P.M. and that was associated with thoughts about how you had nothing to do for the evening. This is your standard schedule these days, but you don't always cut every evening. Do you think there was anything that made you more vulnerable to being home alone with no plans last night? [attempting to identify vulnerability factors that might be open to intervention]

LAURIE: I overheard a couple of colleagues talking earlier in the day about dates they were going on that night and how excited they were. It seemed like they spent hours talking about what they were going to wear. It seemed both totally petty but also sort of enviable.

And then I started thinking about how perfect their lives are, how they don't have any of the same problems as me, that I'm never going to be "normal" like them and it sort of spiraled.

THERAPIST: All this was happening at work? Around what time?

LAURIE: I think it was during my afternoon break that I heard them talking, probably around 3:00ish.

THERAPIST: That sounds really painful and then it also sounds like you heaped a lot of judgments onto it as well. Were you having thoughts about cutting then?

LAURIE: No, I don't think so because I know cutting at work is off-limits for me.

THERAPIST: Any thoughts yet about cutting at home later? Like maybe you knew you weren't going to do it at work but you started planning to do it when you got home?

LAURIE: Hmm. I'm not sure I remember that. I think I was really focused on them and their perfect lives.

A Decision Point

Here, the therapist needs to make a decision for the sake of the chain. Does she label this conversation at work the prompting event for the later problem behavior of cutting? Or does she remain thinking that arriving home from work is the prompting event and overhearing this conversation (and the subsequent thoughts and feelings) were vulnerability factors? As discussed in Chapter 1, it is important for therapists to not overthink this point and instead to focus on being effective in conducting the chain to highlight the sequence of events. Hypothesis testing can help elucidate a bit further as necessary. Specifically, hypothesis testing might involve isolating and manipulating aspects of the chain and noticing the effect. By doing so, the therapist is able to put the spotlight on a key variable in the chain and avoid focusing on details that are less relevant. In this chain, it might look like this:

THERAPIST: Do you think that had you not overheard this conversation at work yesterday that you would have cut last night?

LAURIE: Hmm, probably not. I had been doing pretty well since I hadn't cut in 4 days. I think that conversation kind of threw me into a tailspin.

THERAPIST: This is all so helpful to know. So for the sake of this chain analysis, it actually seems that overhearing this conversation was the prompting event that set off the chain of events that eventually led to you cutting several hours later. Do you see how that seems to be so?

LAURIE: Yeah, I get it.

At this point, the therapist has now drawn two circles on the whiteboard with significant space between them. On the left is the prompting event ("overhearing conversation") and on the right is the target behavior ("cutting"). It looks like Figure 3.2. This chain is taking some time to parse out the details. This amount of detail early on in treatment is necessary in order to fully understand the problem and to be able to make successful inroads at treating it. Interestingly, identification of the prompting event actually changed with assessment, which highlights the critical nature of careful questioning.

Identifying Links

THERAPIST: Now that we have the prompting event defined in a different way, I'm going to ask a similar question. Do you think that there was anything that made you more vulnerable to the effects of hearing that conversation yesterday or would that conversation have led to

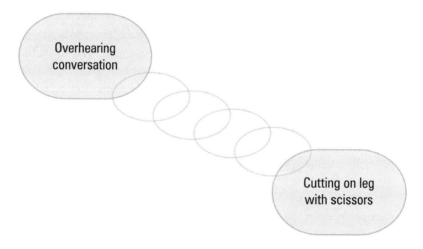

FIGURE 3.2. Chain analysis of Laurie's cutting behavior—start of analysis.

intense emotions no matter what? [Attempting to identify vulnerability factors again in a very specific way. What made the client more vulnerable to the effect of this specific prompting event on this specific day?]

LAURIE: Maybe just feeling more lonely in general lately.

THERAPIST: OK, we'll write down "lonely" here as a vulnerability factor and we'll see what we do with that later as we get more information. Loneliness is a pretty painful feeling and we'll definitely do things to address it as we move forward in treatment; I just want to make sure that we get your cutting under control first. [highlighting target hierarchy and rationale for chain]

LAURIE: OK.

THERAPIST: Now we have a lot of time that elapsed between hearing this conversation around 3:00 and cutting yourself around 10:00. I'd like to first get a sense from you of the general chain of events so that we know what makes sense to zero-in on. Can you just tell me roughly what happened during this time?

The above request for a snapshot overview of what happened is a really useful strategy in cases such as this. If the therapist were to start asking "What happened next? And next? And next?" in an attempt to cover 7 hours of time, this will be the kiss of death for the chain. There will not be enough time in the session and, by session's end, the therapist might only have the first few links of the chain delineated, which might not have the most important information in terms of controlling variables. In addition, it would likely be quite tedious to do and risks disengagement from both parties.

> If there are hours between the prompting event and the problem behavior, first ask the client for a rough overview of what happened during that time to avoid getting bogged down in details.

LAURIE: I stay at work until 5:00, though I have a really hard time concentrating. Feel like I want to cry a lot and I get really short with my customers. I'm sure they all thought I was a bitch-on-wheels or something. I barely even look at Annie and Gina, my colleagues, the rest of the day. At 5:00, I clock out and leave without even saying goodbye! Now I'm feeling really terrible about that too. Why do I have to be such a jerk to everyone?

THERAPIST: Sounds like you are having some guilt or shame about your behavior yesterday? Let's hold on to that—it's going to be another thing that we'll return to—but for now I want to remain focused on yesterday. What were your thoughts and emotions for those couple of hours that you were still at work? Was it sadness? Shame?

LAURIE: I think it was a bit of both and then also some anger. Like "Why do they get to have nice lives while I suffer?"

THERAPIST: Ah, so "It's not fair" showed up?

LAURIE: Yeah, I definitely think those words went through my mind at various points.

THERAPIST: Ok, so for those 2 hours at work, you were feeling a mixture of sadness, shame, and anger, and you were having thoughts that life wasn't fair. You were doing your work but feeling like your mind was elsewhere. Does that seem right?

LAURIE: Yeah, that sounds about right.

THERAPIST: And then you leave work abruptly right at 5:00, without saying goodbye to anyone. During this time, you are not yet thinking about self-injuring in any notable way. Is that correct too?

LAURIE: Yeah.

THERAPIST: OK, so what happens when you leave work?

LAURIE: I remember that when I got into my car, I just felt overwhelmed with sadness. I really didn't want anyone to see me crying in my car so I sort of sped away. I drove to a fast food drive-thru, which is disgusting, but I didn't have anything to eat at home and I couldn't handle going to a store or interacting with anyone. I got a couple of burgers and fries and went home.

THERAPIST: What time did you get home?

LAURIE: I dunno, maybe like 5:45?

THERAPIST: OK, so what happened next? [The therapist is purposely not delving into too many details here because she wants to make sure she gets the "full story" before heading back to parse out more specifics. She is also making a note of all the judgments Laurie is making toward herself and others. This will be important to address but it's the fifth session and the therapist is still trying to understand what's controlling the cutting behavior, so she is not taking the time right now to do more than occasionally observing and labeling the judgments.]

LAURIE: I sat on the couch and ate while watching TV. Just dumb stuff like home improvement shows that I don't have to think too much about.

THERAPIST: I noticed on your diary card that you also drank that night— three beers?—was that at this time?

LAURIE: Yeah, I was drinking beers with dinner. It was not a big deal.

THERAPIST: Maybe not. Over what period of time did you drink those three beers?

LAURIE: Probably about 3 hours. I wasn't even really tipsy.

THERAPIST: OK. Do you think that you would have harmed yourself if you hadn't drank the beers?

LAURIE: Yeah, I don't think the drinking had anything to do with it.

THERAPIST: OK. Let's keep that assumption for now, though we may return to it. So when did urges to self-harm come up?

LAURIE: I don't know. Probably later, like 9:30 or so. I was just getting more and more anxious sitting there on the couch, ruminating over my colleagues and my reaction to it. Like why can't I just be normal and let things go? And it was like this weird combination of boredom and anxiety. I'm not sure I know how to explain it, but it just started growing and growing and I felt like my mind was going berserk and I couldn't control it.

THERAPIST: So this feeling was building up over those few hours? (*Laurie nods.*) And were you doing anything else besides sitting on the couch and watching TV?

LAURIE: No, I felt pretty stuck there in my head.

As of now, the chain that the therapist has drawn on the whiteboard looks like Figure 3.3.

THERAPIST: OK, so what happened around 9:30 when the urge popped up?

LAURIE: Well, like I said, I sort of always have thoughts about cutting in the back of my mind but I was kinda keeping them at bay,

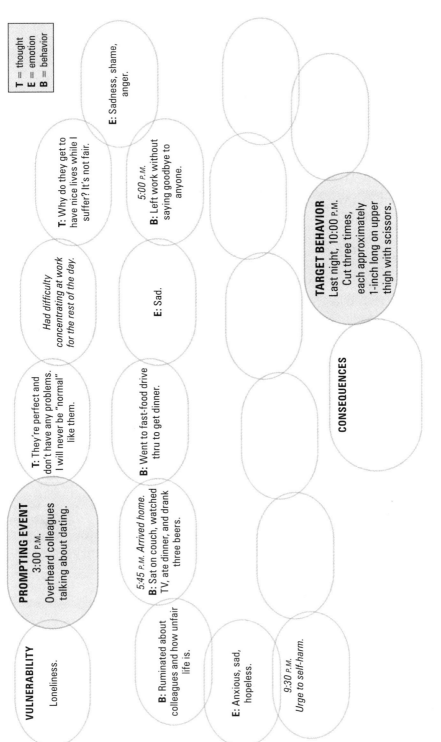

T = thought
E = emotion
B = behavior

VULNERABILITY
Loneliness.

PROMPTING EVENT
3:00 P.M.
Overheard colleagues talking about dating.

T: They're perfect and don't have any problems. I will never be "normal" like them.

Had difficulty concentrating at work for the rest of the day.

T: Why do they get to have nice lives while I suffer? It's not fair.

E: Sadness, shame, anger.

5:45 P.M. Arrived home.
B: Sat on couch, watched TV, ate dinner, and drank three beers.

B: Went to fast-food drive thru to get dinner.

E: Sad.

5:00 P.M.
B: Left work without saying goodbye to anyone.

B: Ruminated about colleagues and how unfair life is.

E: Anxious, sad, hopeless.

9:30 P.M.
Urge to self-harm.

CONSEQUENCES

TARGET BEHAVIOR
Last night, 10:00 P.M.
Cut three times, each approximately 1-inch long on upper thigh with scissors.

FIGURE 3.3. Chain analysis of Laurie's cutting behavior—mid-analysis.

remembering my promise to you and also the fact that I don't have razors in the house anymore.

THERAPIST: That's good. Both of those things are good.

LAURIE: Yeah, but then I just started thinking about it more—how cutting, like nothing else, will reduce my anxiety right away. It would give my brain a break.

THERAPIST: You had those thoughts?

LAURIE: Yeah. and once I thought about that, I knew I was going to do it.

THERAPIST: So let's pause right there. Can you spell that out for me a little bit? I need to know exactly how that happens since it seems so critical.

This is an example of how the therapist homes in for more information if she is not yet clear of how events transpired; if she can't see it in her own mind's eye. In this case, the links probably cover just a minute or two but seem directly relevant to the actual occurrence of the behavior. Since the therapist doesn't quite understand what Laurie is describing here, she asks for more information.

LAURIE: Not sure how well I can describe it. I was sitting there, feeling terrible, like I was glued to the couch even though I wasn't feeling happy there. My head was spinning and the beers and attempt to zone out hadn't done anything to reduce that. I thought about cutting and how cutting always makes me feel better and so I sort of just decided to do it.

THERAPIST: Oh no! Did any other alternatives enter your mind? Either before or after that decision?

LAURIE: Well I thought about calling you, but I actually was angry at that moment at you that you had made me get rid of my razors. I knew you would try to talk me out of it and I didn't want that.

THERAPIST: Oh, so willfulness was there too? Like you remembered the commitment to me and you knew in your wise mind that calling me would likely be effective in getting you to not cut but you became willful about being more skillful?

LAURIE: I wasn't thinking in those terms, but yeah, I guess that's what happened.

THERAPIST: OK, so you actively made the decision "I'm going to cut."

And then what happened? Because of course you could make that decision and still not cut.

LAURIE: *(confused)* Uh, I don't get that really. But I made the decision and then I started thinking about what I could use since I didn't have the razors and I sure as hell wasn't going to leave the house to go to the store.

THERAPIST: And what happened to your anxiety and rumination then?

LAURIE: Huh. I didn't realize it but I think they went away then because I had something else to think about.

THERAPIST: Wow, that is really important! So even thinking and planning for the self-injury reduced your emotional distress a lot.

LAURIE: Yeah.

THERAPIST: I don't think we realized that before in the other assessments we have done.

LAURIE: No, I don't think so either.

THERAPIST: What happened next?

LAURIE: I got up finally and started going through the rooms of my apartment looking for ideas. I thought about using a kitchen knife but for some reason that grossed me out. So stupid really, but I thought that using something that I use to cook with would be too much. Then in my bedroom, I found some scissors that I hadn't used in forever. I took them to the bathroom to clean with antiseptic and then cut myself.

THERAPIST: In the bathroom?

LAURIE: Yeah, I sat down at the edge of the bathtub, pulling up my shorts and did it.

THERAPIST: Like three cuts in quick succession or did you cut and then do something else and cut again?

LAURIE: No, three altogether.

Identifying Consequences

THERAPIST: And what happened next? The immediate consequence of cutting yourself?

LAURIE: I felt really badly that I had done it again.

THERAPIST: Well, wait. Did that happen immediately? Or did those feelings come later?

LAURIE: They seemed to come pretty darn quick, but maybe I had a minute or two of relief. Though I actually think the relief happens as I'm cutting, if that makes sense. And as soon as I'm done, I'm filled with regret.

THERAPIST: I think I get it. It's kind of like you are caught up in the actual activity and are really focused on that. We just need to get you to experience that with behaviors that don't actually hurt you!

LAURIE: Yeah, I guess you're right. I just don't know what those are.

THERAPIST: Before we move on to possible solutions and ways to get this to go differently, are there any other consequences that you can think of? In yourself or in the environment? Did you tell anyone?

LAURIE: No. And I knew I couldn't call you anymore that night.

THERAPIST: Correct. I so wish you had called me earlier.

LAURIE: Yeah, me too. I don't remember anything else that was a consequence. I actually went to bed pretty soon after.

THERAPIST: Do you think that you were able to fall asleep because you weren't as anxious anymore?

LAURIE: Oh, definitely. So maybe it helped with that too.

THERAPIST: Maybe. Though I would prefer to say that having reduced anxiety helped with that, not cutting.

LAURIE: OK, I get your point.

This chain with Laurie took about 40 minutes to complete. At the end, the therapist has written the sequence in Figure 3.4 on the whiteboard. Notice that she does not take the time to write out every single detail because that would likely take up too much time and is likely not necessary.

As in Sasha's chain, this chain illustrates that the process is usually far from tedious. Learning about your client and his or her behavior using the structure of chain analysis can be extraordinarily useful, collaborative, as well as relationship building. The chains for Laurie and Sasha both illustrate assessment of a top target behavior and thus were completed early in treatment. However, later in treatment, a "first chain" may be conducted on a new behavior that has just started occurring (e.g., a client reports that she shoplifted for the first time in the prior week) or on a problem that becomes a new priority, after other problems have been addressed. These chains might look different from the first chain

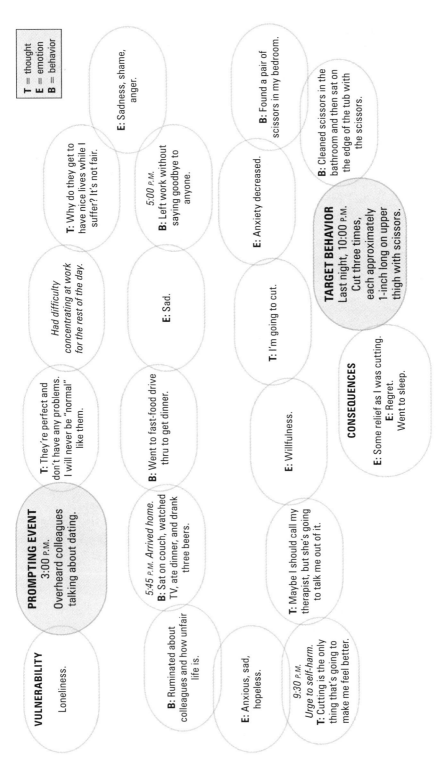

FIGURE 3.4. Chain analysis of Laurie's cutting behavior—complete.

conducted in treatment because the therapist may not have to orient the client to the rationale and process of the assessment. However, the therapist still wants to follow the same principles outlined so far.

Chain Analysis of Isaac's Anger Behavior

Isaac, a 42-year old man, came to treatment initially for help with severe depression, which was associated with staying in bed for hours every day, social isolation, and suicidal ideation. After 3 months of working from a behavioral activation approach, his suicidal ideation had been absent for a full month. While continuing to monitor for depression behaviors, the therapist turned to Isaac's next target for treatment. Isaac stated that he needed help with "anger" and stated that his wife had threatened to leave him unless he got his anger under control. Together, the therapist and Isaac put "anger" on the agenda to assess.

> "You've said that you have problems with anger and yet I don't really know what that means for you. I'd like to spend some time talking about what anger looks like for you, the ways in which it causes problems for you, and even focus in on a recent experience with anger so that I can better understand what it's like for you. Is that OK?"

After asking some questions about Isaac's general experience of anger, the therapist goes on to explore the nature of Isaac's anger by stating that she is interested in focusing on *one* recent experience. In that sense, she is beginning a chain analysis, but I'm going to illustrate a slightly different way of obtaining the information for the chain. In this scenario, the therapist first asks Isaac to give a general description of what happened and then goes back to "fill in" the details of the chain. If the therapist chooses this approach, it remains critical that he or she keep the components of the chain in mind as the focus of the assessment.

THERAPIST: As I said, in order for me to get a good idea of what this anger problem looks like for you, it would help me if we focused on an example of a recent experience with anger that you think illustrates the kind of problems you have. Can you think of one recent occurrence that stands out to you?

ISAAC: Probably last week, when my wife said she would leave if I didn't get help.

THERAPIST: It sounds like that would be a good episode to focus on for many reasons. Do you remember when exactly that was?

ISAAC: Last Tuesday.

THERAPIST: Great. Why don't we start by you just giving me an overview of what happened and then we can go into it in more detail?

ISAAC: Sure. I had come home from work and was just in a pretty crummy mood. It seemed like my wife started criticizing me as soon as I walked in the door—why hadn't I remembered to pick up the dry cleaning, why I had left so many dishes in the sink that morning, that I'm not doing enough to support the family—it just felt like she was dumping everything onto me and not acknowledging her role in anything. And I got really frustrated and was tired of holding everything in and just being her punching bag. So I started to shout back at her and we went back and forth for a while and I just got more and more angry because she wasn't listening to me. So I just picked up the vase from the table and threw it against the wall. And she screamed that she couldn't take it anymore and walked out of the house. She didn't come back until a few hours later and then she told me that if I didn't get help, she was going to leave because she couldn't live with me like this anymore.

THERAPIST: Sounds like a really intense experience. Have you thrown stuff in anger before or was this the first time?

ISAAC: No, unfortunately, not the first time. I don't always throw stuff when I'm angry but it's happened a few times in the past year.

THERAPIST: Do things ever get physical between you and your wife during these fights?

ISAAC: Do I ever hit her? No.

THERAPIST: Do you ever throw things at her?

ISAAC: No, never. I would never do that, I don't think. I have thrown things at the wall or on the floor.

At this point, the therapist has gotten a brief narrative of the event from last week. She has also assessed whether there is any violence in the relationship and will continue to keep an eye out for this behavior.

Although Isaac said he doesn't always throw things when angry, it does sometimes occur and thus we can think of this example as a representative behavior to analyze more fully. Now that the therapist has the overview of the event, she can move into a more structured chain.

Reorienting the Client

THERAPIST: OK, so I now have a little bit of an idea of what happened last Tuesday. Given that anger is what you want to work on, and the fact that this was a pretty serious event, I would like for us to go into it in a bit more detail and do a chain analysis, if that's OK with you. This is similar to the chains we have done in the past on your suicide ideation. Since it's been a little while since we have done a chain analysis, I want to remind you of the reasons for doing them. One is that I want to learn more about it by figuring out all the thoughts and emotions you were having, as well as the sorts of things that made you more vulnerable to this fight happening, and two, I want us to start to identify points in the sequence of events where you could have done something differently to prevent the fight from either occurring at all or escalating to the point where you threw something. How does that sound to you?

ISAAC: Good.

Defining the Target Behavior

THERAPIST: Great, we're on the same page. Just like we've done with other problems before now, I want us to try to understand how the chain of events happened, how all the links in a chain are connected. (*Draws out picture of chain on whiteboard.*) So the first thing we need to do is identify the key problem behavior of this chain. For the time being, I'd like to label throwing the vase as the problem behavior. We might change this later, but for now it gives us a point to focus on.

ISAAC: OK.

THERAPIST: So you picked up a vase from a table and threw it at a wall. Where were you? Can you describe the scene a little bit, as if I was watching this on a movie screen?

ISAAC: Sure, we were in the kitchen, both standing up near the table.

She was moving around, yelling and putting dishes away, not really looking at me. I was so mad and angry that she was criticizing me and also not looking at me and talking to me directly. I just picked up the vase from the center of the table and threw it against the opposite wall. It shattered and the glass, water, and flowers just went everywhere.

THERAPIST: That's really helpful. I think I can picture that. Do you remember what time this was on Tuesday, so that we can anchor it in time a bit?

ISAAC: It was probably just a few minutes after I got home, it all happened so fast, maybe around 6:15?

THERAPIST: And if you were to rate your anger on a scale of 1 to 10 at that moment you threw the vase, what would you say?

ISAAC: A definite 10.

Identifying Consequences

THERAPIST: And what happened immediately after you threw the vase? [assessing consequences]

ISAAC: My wife screamed at me, "What the hell are you doing?," and then said how she couldn't take it anymore, got her bag, and left.

THERAPIST: What happened within you immediately after you threw the vase?

ISAAC: What do you mean?

THERAPIST: I mean, what were you thinking and feeling? Do you remember?

ISAAC: I think I was feeling incredibly frustrated and out of control. I just completely lost it. And when she stormed out, at first I felt good and empowered, but then as time went on I started to just hate myself.

THERAPIST: What do you mean by that? Sounds really painful.

ISAAC: Like, what kind of person am I that I can't control myself at all. This is not who I want to be.

THERAPIST: It sounds to me that your behavior didn't match your values. That's good for me to know and will definitely help us figure out how to change it. What happened to your anger? Did it go down when you threw the vase or hang around longer?

ISAAC: It seemed like it went down but I'm not sure if that was because I threw the vase or because my wife left.

THERAPIST: OK, that's fair. We might not know what caused it to go down but we know that it did. In general, when you've thrown objects in the past, did your anger go down right away?

ISAAC: Hmm, I don't think so. At other times, it's stayed pretty high. Hard to say for sure.

THERAPIST: OK, so let's go back to Tuesday.

The therapist has now assessed the problem behavior and its consequences. In terms of the problem behavior, note that although Isaac said that his problem is "anger," the therapist looked for a problem *behavior* associated with anger. This focus on overt behavior is more clinically useful for a couple of reasons: (1) it provides a more concrete event on which to focus and can be anchored in time; this is opposed to the experience of an emotion, where it is difficult to identify a starting and ending point or the moment it becomes a "problem"; and (2) the problem for Isaac is not the presence of anger itself but of the behaviors associated with it. In other words, the therapist wants to avoid the notion that they're going to work together to get rid of anger as though anger should never be experienced. Instead, the goals are to reduce problem behaviors associated with anger, and reduce the intensity and duration of anger.

This chain shows how sometimes it is more natural to focus on the consequences after the target behavior, instead of first going back to the prompting event. As discussed in Chapter 1, the exact order in which you do the chain is less important than getting the necessary information. The therapist has to keep track of what's been assessed and what information still needs to be gathered, which can be challenging when you're moving back and forth from the general to the specifics. Using a whiteboard or writing the chain out in a collaborative fashion, in addition to keeping the client engaged, also helps the therapist stay on track. Since this is the first chain on this problem, the therapist may also ask other questions about how this experience relates to other similar anger-related behaviors. These types of questions are important in communicating to the client that the therapist is not focused on one event to the point of excluding the rest of his life. A client could feel very dissatisfied with a session if he or she spent the entire time focused on one incident without relating it to the broader problems for which he or she is seeking help. At the same time, the therapist in this example is continuing to orient Isaac as to why she is seeking this information and also continually assessing his willingness to continue with his chain.

Identifying the Prompting Event and Vulnerabilities

Let's say that the therapist and Isaac next identify the prompting event and vulnerabilities. Isaac states that his anger immediately shot up when he walked in the house and the first thing his wife said was, "Why didn't you clean the dishes before you left for work this morning?" This statement by his wife was labeled the prompting event. The therapist next asked if anything made him more vulnerable to his wife's comment on Tuesday. Isaac responded that he had had a difficult day at work and was feeling generally dissatisfied with his career. He also stated that he had slept poorly the night before and woke up late that morning and had to rush to get to work on time. All of those things contributed to him feeling like he was having a "bad day."

Identifying Links

The therapist then moves to the links in the chain between the prompting event (comment by wife) and problem behavior (throwing vase). Isaac had previously stated that it was just a few minutes and that things happened very quickly. Obtaining the exact back-and-forth communication between Isaac and his wife is not relevant here. Instead, a focus on emotions and cognitions as the fight occurs would yield more important information about Isaac that is relevant for understanding not only this exact fight but also how his thinking and emotions are related to the problem behaviors associated with anger more broadly. The links might look like this:

> Comment by wife → *Thought:* "Doesn't she realize there might be valid reasons for why I didn't do those things?" → Disappointment, frustration → Start criticizing back, instead of explaining what happened → Back and forth yelling about the others' faults → Anger increasing → *Thought:* "She doesn't get me at all. She's not listening to what I have to say." → *Statement:* "Just turn around and look at me, you're being a b—!" → Wife does not turn around and her angry comments escalate → *Thought:* "I'll make her look at me!" → Looks around for something to throw and spots vase on table → Throws vase.

Now we have a complete assessment of Isaac's anger episode culminating in him throwing the vase and his wife leaving for several hours. The order in which the information was obtained varied from Sasha's and Laurie's chains but the end result is the same. The therapist has an idea of how this behavior came to occur, can see the event in her "mind's eye," and has begun to identify potential points that will require more assessment. For example, the therapist may need to know a bit more about the nature of Isaac and his wife's relationship in order to better understand why the comment by his wife affected him so strongly. (It's not that his reaction wasn't understandable; it's that some people might hear that comment and more easily brush it off). The therapist might also want to assess Isaac's relationship history, especially in his family of origin, to better understand the role of anger in his relationships and the ways in which anger behavior may have been modeled or reinforced. Furthermore, Isaac discussed how he is not feeling good at his job and this might be an area of further assessment as well since it's quite possible that his anger episodes are directly tied to broader feelings of dissatisfaction with his life. Ultimately, this highly structured assessment yielded an abundance of information that will be useful for solution analysis and generation purposes.

In this chapter, I discussed what chain analyses might look like when assessing a problem behavior for the first time, whether it occurs in an early treatment session or later in therapy after other problems have been addressed. I provided three examples of different types of target behaviors. Each of these examples illustrated how the five components of the chain can be elicited as well as how orienting comments can be woven into the chain. Further, they each demonstrate that such fine-grained assessment of key target behaviors can be a rich clinical exercise yielding a lot of information about the behavior as well as the client's life more generally. In spite of this, the process of assessment is not always smooth, so now we turn next to discussion of how to keep clients engaged throughout chain analyses.

CHAPTER 4

Keeping the Client Engaged (and You Too!)

A frequent challenge in conducting chain analyses is keeping clients and therapists engaged in the task. There is a misconception that this part of therapy is dry, but when done well and with purpose that is far from the truth. This chapter is all about how to incorporate validation, stylistic, and dialectical strategies into the basics of chains to enliven the process, keep commitment strong, and increase effectiveness. Examples with various choice points will be presented to show how different strategies can have demonstrable effects on the outcome of the analysis. These strategies are important in chains when first assessing behavior, like those described in the previous chapter, as well as in repeated chains when behaviors aren't changing and the therapist needs to conduct more assessment to determine what's missing (to be discussed in Chapter 6). Together, these strategies help the therapist and the client stay engaged, and therefore make it a more compelling exercise.

Validation Strategies in Chain Analysis

If you have been conducting DBT, you are likely familiar with the importance of validation in the treatment. Along with behaviorism and dialectics, validation is one of the three core sets of strategies that are the foundation of DBT. Chain analysis, the process by which behavioral assessment is conducted, falls under the "behaviorism" umbrella in DBT, yet dialectics and validation play a critical role in keeping the analysis moving forward in productive ways. There already exist some excellent writings on the broader use of validation in DBT beyond the original treatment manual (see, e.g., Koerner, 2011; Swenson, 2016), and so this discussion will be limited to the ways in which validation strategies can be explicitly woven into the chain analysis.

Validation is used to balance and enhance the change strategies. Linehan (1993) incorporated validation and acceptance into DBT because change strategies alone were not working. That is, she discovered that when she pushed for change in isolation, clients often felt "unheard," and misunderstood. Their experience was that she could not possibly understand the depths of their problems if she was so confident that "simple" behavioral solutions, such as skills, would work at ameliorating them. They also felt that she was replicating their previous experiences with caregivers who invalidated their intense emotional experiences by suggesting that their problems were easily solved or that they should just "get over" them. Such feedback led to the incorporation of validation into the broader treatment to communicate understanding, acceptance, and empathy. It allowed the client to feel fully understood, and therefore more willing to go along with the change strategies that the therapist suggested.

Validation is especially relevant for chains because a primary function of validation is to help with the change process. Metaphorically, validation is the grease that keeps the wheels of change moving; it is not the movement of the wheels. It is also possible to overdo validation in a couple of notable ways: (1) if a therapist is overly focused on validation, a client may feel understood but not helped; and (2) if a client is effectively working on a problem with a therapist, too much validation can actually derail the process. Too much grease on the wheels can cause them to slip. In fact, Linehan has described what happened when she swung too far in the direction of validation (Linehan & Wilkes, 2015). She found that by focusing entirely on validation, clients still felt invalidated because she wasn't doing anything to help them change the situations that caused them so much suffering. It may take some time to determine what the right balance is for any given client across multiple circumstances; however, even without knowing the client that well, it is important for the therapist to keep *balance* in mind.

> Validation is used to balance and enhance the change strategies that comprise chain analysis.

Let's return to the client Sasha discussed in the last chapter. The chain of her drinking behavior was moving along at a steady clip and the therapist was assessing the links between the prompting event and the target behavior. He got to the point where Sasha was describing the argument with her boyfriend and she said that they "hashed out all the things we hate about each other" and during this fight, she reported feeling intense anger, shame, and sadness. Imagine the therapist did this:

THERAPIST: Wow, this must have been a very painful fight for you.

SASHA: Yeah, it was. (*Starts looking down, gets quiet.*)

THERAPIST: I can imagine why—here you two were, saying all these things to each other that were hurtful.

SASHA: Mmm-hmm.

THERAPIST: If I were in that experience, I would feel the same way.

SASHA: (*Nods.*)

THERAPIST: And now I'm making you talk about all this again, which is bringing up those difficult feelings for you all over again!

SASHA: (*silence*)

In this scenario, each time the therapist spoke, he attempted to validate Sasha by highlighting the difficulty of the experience and the emotions she expressed. However, this focus on validation leads to Sasha's becoming less active in the session and potentially shutting down. It is possible that by highlighting the pain and difficult emotions, Sasha begins to also experience hopelessness. One can picture her thinking (though not expressing) something like, "This is all so difficult; it's never going to change." The validation here may help Sasha feel the therapist gets what happened but it does not express that the therapist knows what's needed to get things to change.

I can imagine that some readers might be thinking, "What's so wrong with this scenario? Don't we want clients to experience emotions in session and for the therapist to allow emotional expression? Wouldn't redirecting her to the chain be invalidating?" My answer to this, as is my answer to so many DBT-related questions, is "It depends"! One might imagine a scenario later in treatment, after a client's behavior is assessed with multiple chains, when a therapist begins to identify a pattern of shutting down in the face of extreme emotions, which interferes with problem solving. Such a pattern might be identified as an important problem and addressed in a multitude of ways. However, remember that this chain with Sasha was the first she engaged in; the therapist's goal is to complete the chain and have it be an overall fruitful experience. A therapist can validate the pain and difficulty without overdoing it. This can be accomplished in the following way:

THERAPIST: Wow, this must have been a very painful fight for you.

SASHA: Yeah, it was. (*Starts looking down, gets quiet.*)

THERAPIST: It seems to me like this is all the more reason to really under-stand what happened and how this led to you drinking. It may be that we come back and see how we prevent these fights from occur-ring in the first place, or how to keep them from escalating to such a hurtful point. And, in order for that to happen, we need to get you to stop drinking. So can we go back to what happened after the fight?

SASHA: Yeah, I suppose. (*Sits up a bit in her chair.*)

In this scenario, the therapist still validates and then redirects back to the chain. He redirects in a way that highlights possible solutions as well as orienting to the task at hand. In so doing, he also likely prevents Sasha from shutting down, which is important for using the session time to make progress on this key target. In fact, we could label the therapist behavior as an instance of "functional validation" (Linehan, 1997) in which the therapist responds to the behavior as something that is serious and worth attention, and, by so doing, validates the importance of this problem and therefore the importance of solving the problem.

However, there are other scenarios in which a lot of validation may be necessary in order to achieve collaboration in the process of chain analysis. Such scenarios may be punctuated by a client's willfulness about discussing a behavior in depth or extreme emotions that interfere with the process of discussing links in the chain. In the first couple of chains, it is often not clear to what extent a behavior that shows up during a chain (e.g., willfulness) is representative of a pattern. In these early chains, the therapist might have to rely more on validation to keep the chain going than he or she would in later chains when patterns are identified, labeled, and treated in other ways.

In summary, the therapist wants to strategically use validation dur-ing a chain analysis to communicate understanding and acceptance of the client and his or her behavior. In the context of the chain, validation serves to keep the client motivated to continue with the process of the assessment, and, ultimately, in solving the problem. The therapist uses validation to achieve collaboration with the recognition that more validation is not always better validation.

Stylistic Strategies: Balancing Reciprocal Communication and Irreverence

In addition to incorporating validation into chains, it is often helpful to mindfully integrate stylistic strategies. The stylistic strategies in DBT refer to the style and form with which the therapist delivers the treatment including chain analyses. A DBT therapist strives to dialectically balance *responsive communication* and *irreverent communication*. Responsive communication involves warmth, reciprocal communication, genuineness, self-disclosure, and taking the client and his or her problems seriously. In contrast, irreverent communication is designed to catch the client off-guard and to stimulate a new way of thinking. Strategies for irreverence include being matter-of-fact and blunt, using a deadpan style, reframing what the client says in an unorthodox or surprising manner, plunging in "where angels fear to tread," directly confronting maladaptive behavior, using humor, oscillating intensity, and assuming both omnipotence and impotence. Going back and forth between these two styles is an essential component of adherent DBT and functions to keep the client engaged, interested, and "awake" to shifts and changes. Vacillation of styles contributes to a sense of movement during sessions.

In the process of a chain, a multitude of opportunities arise to incorporate styles of both reciprocal communication and irreverence. In my opinion, a chain is likely to go much better and maintain both parties' interest if the therapist alternates between the two rather than overly focus on one approach. Reciprocal communication is necessary to convey warmth and care and protects the therapist from coming across as overly technical or rigid in the chain. Irreverence helps to keep the clients' attention and frequently helps them talk about topics they would otherwise want to avoid. In my experience teaching DBT to students and practitioners, therapists often have greater problems learning how to incorporate irreverence into chains than responsive communication, which comes more naturally to them (or has been trained in them for longer). They fear being perceived as overly blunt, mean, or sarcastic, and so they hold back from even trying an irreverent strategy. However, this often leads to missed opportunities to get the client's attention in a way that forces him or her back to the present moment with perhaps a new way of looking at the problem.

Both irreverence and reciprocal communication can occur in verbal and nonverbal forms and do not need to take up significant time in order to be effective. Sometimes a quick facial expression alone is irreverent. A look of shock (raised eyebrows, eyes wide, mouth open) in response to a client talking about an extremely dysfunctional behavior might convey a "You did *what?*" communication without uttering a word. In contrast, a therapist can adopt a very caring expression and lean forward in his or her chair to demonstrate that he or she is totally and completely there for the client in a warm and accepting manner. Similarly, a short phrase might provide an irreverent jolt to the interaction or balance out an otherwise warm and validating interaction. For example, in the midst of discussing a problem behavior, a therapist might pause and state in an intense and incredulous manner, "Let me get this straight—you started thinking about death and causing harm to yourself because you were too cold in bed and couldn't figure out how to solve the problem?!?" In this way, irreverence can frequently function to invalidate the invalid by essentially communicating "This is ineffective. There may be valid aspects to what you did/thought/felt but ultimately there are way more effective responses to the situation."

It is important to recognize that, similarly to validation, it is possible to overdo one form of stylistic communication. Too much reciprocal communication in the absence of irreverence can lead to slow sessions that don't progress much and are bogged down by a sort of excess empathy. Too much irreverent communication leads to the loss of impact of any one irreverent communication. If irreverence functions to get a client's attention but all the therapist does is attempt to use irreverence, it ceases to do its job. Thus, it is vital for therapists to keep these strategies in a dialectical balance as well. In the context of chain analyses, a therapist may wonder to what extent a balance of stylistic communication is necessary. I would argue that they are just as important here as in any other aspect of the treatment in order to keep the client engaged and interested, as well as to ultimately help shape them toward engaging in more effective behavior.

Many stylistic strategies use nonverbal communication or tone of voice, which are difficult to portray in written form. However, I'd like to show what each side could look like in a series of vignettes from the case of Belinda, a 20-year-old woman living at home with her mother. Due to a pattern of unrelenting crisis and severe depression, Belinda spent most of her time at home isolated in her bedroom. The chain in these vignettes occurred following an episode in which Belinda got in a fight with her mother (prompting event) about how her cat made a mess of her cat food and Belinda did not clean it up. A few minutes later, Belinda went to her room and tightened a belt around her neck (target behavior).

Vignette 1: Therapist Unbalanced in Favor of Reciprocal Communication during Chain Analysis

THERAPIST: So you got to your room and put the belt around your neck. How did you feel just prior to that—what emotions were you experiencing?

BELINDA: I just felt really hopeless about everything—whether my relationship with my mother could ever change, whether I'll ever be able to live independently and not have to deal with all this crap.

THERAPIST: That sounds so painful. I would be upset over the fight too. (warm, soothing voice tone) [disclosure aiming to normalize client reaction] So then what happened?

BELINDA: I saw a belt lying on the floor and just started to wonder what it would feel like around my neck—whether I could be brave enough to pull it tight.

THERAPIST: So you were thinking that this would be a way to get rid of your bad feelings? [validation]

BELINDA: Yeah, it seemed like the only thing to do.

THERAPIST: It sounds like you were feeling really hopeless. (warm tone) [taking problems seriously, validation] What happened after you had put the belt around your neck?

BELINDA: A mixture of things, I guess. I was no longer thinking about the fight but I also wasn't feeling good about what I was doing.

THERAPIST: Ah. So a consequence of this behavior was that it helped reduce the distress of the fight. Am I getting that right? [checking in with client]

In this very short vignette, the therapist was keeping the chain moving forward while, stylistically speaking, maintaining a purely reciprocal stance. Thus, in some senses, this is a fine chain in that the assessment function was still being met, the client was participating, and the chain was progressing. However, there are risks associated with being imbalanced in favor of reciprocal communication, especially if the entire chain was conducted in this manner. One risk is that the chain may lack a sense of movement, speed, and flow and appear relatively tedious without anything capturing the client's attention. Thus, the client's level of engagement may start to suffer over time. A second risk is that, although the client was responding to the validation, a therapist that is overly reciprocal runs the risk of functionally validating "invalid" behavior. That is, by not "calling out" a client on his or her dysfunctional behavior or the maladaptive links in the chain, the therapist might be tacitly agreeing that it all made sense and was normative. Let's see what this same scenario might look like if irreverence is incorporated into the process of the chain.

Vignette 2: Therapist Integrating Irreverence into Chain of Dysfunctional Behavior

THERAPIST: So you got to your room and put the belt around your neck. How did you feel just prior to that—what emotions were you experiencing?

BELINDA: I just felt really hopeless about everything—whether my relationship with my mother could ever change, whether I'll ever be able to live independently and not have to deal with all this crap.

THERAPIST: So then what happened?

BELINDA: I saw a belt lying on the floor and just started to wonder what it would feel like around my neck—whether I could be brave enough to pull it tight.

THERAPIST: So wait. Let me get this straight because I'm really confused. *(incredulous voice tone, plunging in where angels fear to tread)* A fight about cat food led you to put a belt around your neck??

BELINDA: *(taken aback)* Well, it wasn't just the cat food, it was everything.

THERAPIST: I get that. The cat food fight was kind of representative of all the things you don't like about your current situation, right?

[recripocal—taking client's behavior seriously, warmer tone, and also keeping an irreverent aspect by labeling the prompting event "the cat food fight"]

BELINDA: Right.

THERAPIST: But I hope you can also see how you kind of went along with your thoughts and urges as though you were on autopilot. As though this all made complete sense as a thing to do in response to the situation that started with a fight about cat food. [confronting]

BELINDA: Yeah, I guess. But my mother was being so rude to me!

THERAPIST: So *that* justifies putting a belt around your neck? Your mother was rude?! If I did something like that every time someone was rude to me, I would be covered in black and blue marks! [reframing in unorthodox manner; intense style]

BELINDA: OK, OK! I get your point. Now what?

THERAPIST: Listen *(shifting to warm voice tone)*, I'm on your side here. I just want you to realize that autopilot is not your friend right now because you start to think that all your responses make sense, given the situation, instead of seeing all the alternatives that are available. Which is all the more reason why we have to unpack this further and figure out all the links that got you from A to B so that we can also figure out what needs to be different.

In this scenario, the therapist continues to conduct the chain in a manner that keeps the assessment moving and yet does not hesitate to point out dysfunctional behaviors along the way. By alternating between irreverence and reciprocal communication, the therapist keeps the client engaged, aware, and on her toes. The therapist is careful not to go too far in one direction so that the client does not just go along on "autopilot" nor does she feel invalidated, which runs the risk of decreased participation and collaboration.

> Alternate between irreverence and reciprocal communication, to keep the client engaged, aware, and on her toes but be careful not to become imbalanced in one direction.

In summary, the stylistic communication strategies are extremely useful tools available to the therapist during chain analyses. It is important for therapists to expand their own repertoires to include both irreverent and reciprocal strategies even if it is initially outside their comfort zone. By doing so, the chain analyses are likely to be more productive.

Dialectical Strategies in Chain Analysis

Dialectical philosophy is a core foundation of DBT and is found throughout all aspects of treatment. To briefly review, the dialectical worldview posits that everything (and everyone) is connected and in constant change. These connections and changes produce tensions and polarities that are both unavoidable and necessary. A dialectical worldview suggests that from these tensions and polarities, new syntheses are born, which, in time, produce their own antitheses. An important tenet of dialectical philosophy, especially in the context of chain analyses, is that there is no absolute truth. That is, neither the client nor the therapist has a "lock" on the truth and what's right. Thus, assessment serves a vital role in trying to determine "what is being left out" of any one person's understanding of the problem and its causes and consequences.

A DBT therapist models a dialectical worldview whenever possible and uses specific dialectical strategies throughout sessions. Although the primary dialectic in DBT treatment is to effectively balance acceptance and change strategies, there are also specific dialectical strategies that are meant to assist the therapist when polarization or "stuckness" arises in treatment. In the context of a chain, examples of polarization could include those shown in Table 4.1.

TABLE 4.1. Examples of Polarizations in Chain Analysis

CLIENT: I don't want to talk about this.	↔	THERAPIST: You have to talk about this if you want things to be different.
CLIENT: I know what the problem is and it's [just one specific aspect of chain]. I don't need to talk about anything else.	↔	THERAPIST: The problem is way more than just that one specific aspect and we need to talk about all of it if we're going to make a difference.
CLIENT: We don't have to talk about this problem anymore since I've already resolved not to do it again	↔	THERAPIST: A simple resolution won't work; we have to analyze the problem in detail in order to get it to stop.

Specific dialectical strategies are briefly described in Table 4.2. A therapist could incorporate one of them, as needed, into the chain analysis when the analysis gets stuck. However, even without thinking of these specific strategies (and in moments of high tension in therapy, it may be difficult to remember them), if a therapist learns to become more attentive to moments of polarization, just observing and describing it can be very helpful. Modeling dialectical thinking is a dialectical strategy in itself and can be incredibly useful in letting the client in on the workings of the therapist's brain. For example, a therapist might say, "I'm noticing that there's a potential conflict here. You believe that talking about this problem in detail in a chain is not necessary since you've already resolved not to do it again and I believe that doing a chain on the behavior is the only way to learn how to get it to not occur again. There's truth on both sides. I wonder what we might do to get to the middle, the synthesis." Sometimes the therapist feels like he or she needs to know what the synthesis *is* before broaching the topic of dialectical tension. However, that is likely a nondialectical approach to the problem! Further, the client can often generate a synthesis that the therapist would never think of.

One of the biggest obstacles to using dialectical strategies during chains is the therapist not realizing that there is polarization. This can happen for a number of reasons including the therapist believing that he or she already knows the "right" answers and moves forward with only his or her own assumptions or the therapist plows on with the chain despite the lack of participation from the client. The lack of awareness could also occur because there are more subtle forms of polarization when the tension between the therapist and the client is not so evident. For example, a client could become less responsive over time and not detail reasons for why that is so. It could also be that the therapist believes that the client is on board with what they're trying to accomplish when in fact the client has had a change of mind and does not express this change to the therapist.

> Incorporate a dialectical strategy into the chain when the analysis gets stuck, usually because of polarization.

So how does the therapist become more aware of polarization during a chain and therefore when dialectical strategies are needed? Tactics for becoming more aware range in degrees of effort involved. For example, therapists can record therapy sessions and watch them to identify

TABLE 4.2. Relevant Dialectical Strategies for Polarization in Chain Analyses

Strategy	Brief description
Enter the paradox	Therapist highlights the contradictions of client's behavior or argument, or reality in general. *Example:* "The more you don't want to talk about this problem, the more crucial it is to discuss."
Use metaphors/ stories	Therapist uses a metaphor or story to describe what is being discussed in therapy in more relatable terms. *Example:* "You cutting yourself in the midst of huge distress and yet refusing to do a chain is like a person who's drowning refusing to take the life preserver thrown to him."
Play devil's advocate	Therapist takes an extreme oppositional perspective in order to get the client to argue for a more middle path solution him- or herself. *Example:* "Maybe we shouldn't do a chain—it's going to be too hard. I mean why bother understanding this behavior at all?"
Extending	Therapist extends the implications of the client's communication (used especially when client is speaking from "emotion mind"). *Example:* "Yes, you're right, we should *never* talk about something after it's over. There's nothing to learn *at all* from past events, right?"
Activate "wise mind"	Therapist helps client elicit the wise mind response for the situation in an effort to move from a less extreme position. *Example:* "Sounds like emotion mind is telling you to avoid talking about this right now. What does your wise mind say? Let's take a minute, attend to our breath, and see if wise mind has an opinion here."
Make lemonade out of lemons	Therapist highlights a benefit to the problem or situation that is being discussed. *Example:* "The good news about your drug use this week is that it gives us an opportunity to find out about all the factors related to your use that we would never get otherwise. This is perfect for helping us figure out how to get you to not use again."
Dialectical assessment	Therapist assesses by examining both client's behavior and context for an understanding; therapist constantly asks "What is being left out" of the existing conceptualization of a problem. There is no one sentence or phrase that embodies dialectical assessment—rather it is the frame in which all assessment, and chain analyses, are conducted.

problematic spots from a more objective stance. Therapists can utilize their teams to talk about the lack of progress or movement and specifically ask the team to help them assess whether polarization is a problem. One less effortful strategy that my team has found helpful is to use personal frustration, feelings of stuckness or boredom, and/or feeling as though you are having an argument rather than a discussion as cues that polarization is likely present. Once a cue is present, the therapist can utilize the mindfulness skills of observe and describe to help move forward. First, one needs to notice or observe the cues described above arising within the session. Second, the therapist can describe what he or she is noticing. For example, the therapist could say, "It doesn't seem like you're with me here, and I have the sense that we're not on the same page. Does that feel true to you?" There have been many times in treatment when I have irreverently said to my client, "Are we fighting here? It feels like we're fighting. What's happening?" The goal of identifying polarization and using dialectical strategies is not necessarily to completely solve the problem that's causing an impasse. One needs to recognize that dialectics involves a *process* that itself is constantly changing. Thus, what serves as an impasse in one particular session (e.g., the client does not think that smoking pot is a problem that she wants to work on despite it being on the top of the therapist's target list) may not be an impasse in the subsequent session (e.g., the client comes in and says "I've decided I want to stop smoking marijuana altogether; it's ruining my life!"). This itself is the nature of dialectics.

Putting It All Together: A Clinical Example

The following example demonstrates how validation, stylistic, and dialectical strategies can be woven into chains. The client, Steve, is a 22-year-old African American man who engages in self-injurious behaviors, often in the form of burning his skin. He has a history of substance use but has been sober for the past 6 months. Self-injurious behavior has been a top target of treatment. The following represents a chain analysis of a recent episode of self-injury (target behavior) early in treatment. It occurred after Steve left his college graduation ceremony abruptly.

THERAPIST: Let's do a chain on what happened with this self-injury.
STEVE: I'm not sure that's what's important.

THERAPIST: What do you mean?

STEVE: Well the burning was because of a bigger issue of me having this embarrassing thing happen at my graduation.

THERAPIST: Oh, and so you're thinking that it's more important to focus on the graduation than the suicidal thoughts specifically? [validating—reflecting back]

STEVE: Yeah, I'm so angry about this so-called friend.

THERAPIST: OK, well the good news is that as we work on the chain for the self-injury, we'll definitely also talk about what happened with your friend since it sounds like an important link on the chain. [Making lemonade out of lemons while staying focused on the priority of the chain. The therapist specifically chose to not validate the emotion here because she did not want the chain to be derailed.] I'd really like to start with the self-injury, though, so that we can figure out how to get that to go away even when you are in difficult situations. OK?

STEVE: OK, fine.

THERAPIST: Great! I know this is not easy and I appreciate your willingness. [validating difficulty of task and praising collaboration] So I know you burned yourself. What did you do exactly and where were you?

STEVE: I was in my car, smoking a cigarette to calm down and then I just took the lit cigarette and pushed it into my arm.

THERAPIST: All right. Can I see where? [irreverence: matter-of-fact tone]

STEVE: *(Pulls up sleeve and shows therapist burn mark on left forearm.)*

THERAPIST: How long do you think you held the cigarette there?

STEVE: I don't know. Probably about 5 seconds or so. I had to feel pain for a bit before it felt like enough.

THERAPIST: *(eyebrows raised, leans forward in chair—both serving to increase intensity)* What do you mean by "enough"?

STEVE: Well, like enough to reduce my emotional pain. It only helped for a little bit though.

THERAPIST: So you're saying it helped you feel better?

STEVE: Yeah.

THERAPIST: You felt better. Damn! It worked. That is the worst news I've heard yet! [irreverence: unorthodox reframe]

STEVE: Yeah. I knew you wouldn't like that. [attentive]

THERAPIST: Well, the good news is that you have me as your therapist because I can get us to figure this out completely. [warm tone as well as omnipotence] Any other consequences? What happened right after?

STEVE: It helped for a few minutes. But then as I was driving home, I just felt crummy again and now maybe even somewhat worse because I was also regretting that I had burned myself after telling you I wouldn't.

THERAPIST: And I just really want to say that I'm so appreciative of you being so honest with me. It really shows me that you're willing to work on difficult things, which is exactly what we need right now. [responsive communication—genuineness and taking client problems seriously]

Commentary

At this point, the therapist has assessed the problem behavior (i.e., self-injury in the form of burning on his left forearm with a lit cigarette) and some immediate consequences subsequent to the self-injury. The therapist has woven in validation in some instances but does not overdo its use. Similarly, at a moment of impasse (Steve saying he didn't want to talk about self-injury per se), the therapist utilized a dialectical strategy to get Steve to move away from his polarized position toward greater willingness. Finally, the therapist has used both reciprocal communication and irreverent styles to keep Steve engaged as well as to get his attention when necessary. Returning to the chain, we'll see the therapist continue to use all these strategies as she assesses the other elements of the chain.

THERAPIST: So now let's go backward: what happened that led to you leaving your graduation and ultimately harming yourself?

STEVE: I had to stand up on a stage in front of a huge projector screen that had pictures of me on it.

THERAPIST: Wow! That sounds intense—did everyone have to do that or was there a reason you specifically did?

STEVE: I was being recognized for an award I got for best paper or something. (*Looks down, visibly embarrassed.*)

THERAPIST: Hmm, I'm noticing that you didn't exactly say that with pride. [irreverence by using playful tone and gentle chiding]

STEVE: No, the whole thing just really embarrassed me.

THERAPIST: OK, we'll have to come back to that at some point later. Doesn't make a whole lot of sense to me right now that winning an award would lead to you harming yourself a short while later. [irreverence: pointing out absence of logic] Go on.

STEVE: And I didn't have a speech because I just didn't.

THERAPIST: Oh dear! Did you know you were expected to make a speech?

STEVE: Well it was all really informal, a small-group graduation. I didn't know that I was going to be called to the podium—I thought I would just have to stand up or something.

THERAPIST: Yikes. I can imagine feeling a lot of stress then when they called you to the podium. That's how I would feel! [validation by normalizing the emotional experience]

STEVE: Totally. So I just sort of mumbled something, I can't even really remember what. And then my friend Rachel gave a speech about me that was semitrue.

THERAPIST: What do you mean "semitrue"?

STEVE: She was just saying random stuff about me and acting like a close friend but she doesn't really know me, so it just felt weird.

THERAPIST: What were you thinking and feeling while you were listening to Rachel?

STEVE: I think it just reminded me of our weird friendship. It was a reminder of things from the past. It felt like really awkward and fake. It just felt really fake.

THERAPIST: So you had the thought "This feels fake." You're feeling awkward, right? I'm still really curious about how this leads to you harming yourself. Were thoughts of self-harm going through your mind then, while you were on stage?

STEVE: I don't really know. It was sort of a lot of stuff going on at once. I don't remember all the *specifics*. (*Appears frustrated, starts looking down at hands.*) This is tedious.

THERAPIST: (*Sits up straighter, raises voice.*) What?!? What could be less tedious than figuring out what causes you to purposely do physical harm to yourself? This seems like life and death to me!

STEVE: *(Looks up, surprised.)* OK! OK! What were you asking?

THERAPIST: Listen, I know I'm asking a lot of detailed questions. This is hard work! We're trying to understand and break a pattern that's been happening within you for years so this won't be easy. I was asking whether you had any urges to self-harm yet when you were on stage at graduation. [Exuding warmth (responsive communication) and validation of difficulty of task]

Commentary

The therapist notes the beginning of the client shutting down and also a possible point of polarization (i.e., the therapist wants to do the chain, but the client does not want to do the chain). Thus, she calls on irreverence, specifically reframing in an unorthodox manner and oscillating intensity to highlight importance and to "wake the client up." Note how in the next statement, she returns to responsive communication by providing a rationale and validating the difficulty of the task. In this way, she demonstrates how a therapist can artfully move on from an irreverent statement in a compassionate manner.

STEVE: No, not specifically. I think I just wanted to escape the whole situation.

THERAPIST: OK, so urges are not on the scene yet. I want to get to that. What else is going on while you're up there on stage?

STEVE: I guess I was feeling angry too.

THERAPIST: What were you angry at?

STEVE: I guess I just felt judged.

THERAPIST: Oh. So you had the thought "People are judging me." What made you feel judged?

STEVE: It's just this beefy white dude culture. We lift weights. We live in the suburbs. It just felt, I don't know. And there were particular people there that I have had interactions with where it felt, I don't know. It just feels uncomfortable. I honestly feel uncomfortable when I'm in a crowd of white people.

THERAPIST: What about it is uncomfortable?

STEVE: I guess sometimes I feel I notice that I stick out or something. I don't know. I'm different.

THERAPIST: That makes a lot of sense. So you were feeling your blackness was more pronounced. [validation]

STEVE: Yeah, even though some people don't even notice it. You don't even notice it.

THERAPIST: *(feeling blindsided)* What do you mean?

STEVE: Well, you can't possibly know what it's like to be black.

THERAPIST: *(pause)* Well, that is totally true. You're exactly right about that. [genuineness] *(pause)* I'm confused though—what's causing you to bring that up now? [irreverence: plunging in where angels fear to tread when therapist would rather avoid this topic entirely]

STEVE: *(getting angry)* I don't know! I'm just so frustrated by it all—all this white privilege everywhere. I can't take it anymore!

THERAPIST: I hear you. The problem is that racism exists in so many different ways in our society and you have to struggle with that on a daily basis. I don't know what that's like personally nor do I know how to completely overcome it. [validation of client's experience] At the same time, learning how to effectively deal with racism when it does occur is unfortunately necessary for survival for you. And as much as I would like for this to be different, I don't think just talking about it will make it go away, do you?

Commentary

Every once in a while (perhaps more often than we care to admit), a therapist is taken off guard by a client's comment rather than the other way around! In this case, the therapist was not expecting to be accused of not understanding something, specifically not understanding the essence of Steve's experience as a black male and the racism he experiences. For many people, when they are accused of "not getting" something, there could be an instant urge to defend ("Of course, I get it!") for fear of otherwise having to admit a weakness or failure or because the associated emotions that the accusation elicits are too painful and the therapist wants to avoid them. This is usually a perfect opportunity for the therapist to make note of his or her own feelings and think strategically about how to use validation, dialectics, and styles to communicate effectively in order to avoid polarization or excessive deviation from the chain. In this example, the therapist pauses before immediately responding, which gives her a chance to check in with herself and what Steve just said. That allows her to have a genuine and honest response—"That is totally true." However, she also continues on by confronting the issue head on in terms of the function of that statement at that moment in the chain analysis. In that sense, she is also keeping the entire chain in mind and remembering her mission during this part of the session.

STEVE: *(Takes a deep breath.)* I know you're right. That doesn't make it easy.

THERAPIST: That is totally true. This is not easy at all. I hope that I'm not giving the impression that it is. [validation, genuineness]

STEVE: You aren't. I just get so frustrated sometimes.

THERAPIST: I don't blame you. I would too. Was the frustration that you're feeling right now similar to what you were feeling at graduation? [stays rooted in the chain]

STEVE: It was worse at graduation I think because I wasn't expressing it—I was just keeping it bottled up inside.

THERAPIST: Ah, OK, that is useful information—when you don't have an outlet, it feels more intense?

STEVE: Yeah.

THERAPIST: And are you, by chance, experiencing any urges to self-harm right now?

STEVE: *(surprised)* No. I wasn't thinking about it.

THERAPIST: Hmm, so even though frustration is present now, there is no urge to self-harm. So there has to be something else that happened at graduation besides frustration about racism, as big as that is, right?

STEVE: Yeah, I guess so. I'm not sure what exactly though.

THERAPIST: Well, let's get back to the chain, and we'll see what we find out. [responsive communication—collaborative language]

STEVE: OK.

THERAPIST: I really appreciate you staying with this—I know it is so hard. So, getting back, you had thoughts, "There are so many white people here and they are judging me." And you were noticing your otherness. Did you have any emotions attached to this?

STEVE: Anger. But also sad too.

THERAPIST: Did you feel shame?

STEVE: Definitely.

THERAPIST: So you were having a lot of emotions. This sounds really difficult. This is why I like to do chain analyses because now I'm starting to understand how you might get to self-harm, though not fully still. It's different than, "I thought this graduation was stupid so I wanted to burn myself." There is so much more to it than that. It's having this shame reaction to these thoughts. So you're on stage and you feel like you're highlighted and the spotlight is on you, so what makes you feel like you have to leave?

STEVE: Well I felt like leaving pretty soon after I got there. I was like, "Holy shit, I really want to leave," less than 5 minutes in.

THERAPIST: Because these thoughts were coming up right away?

STEVE: As soon as they called me to the stage, yeah.

THERAPIST: OK, so we're going to come back to this point for solutions in a bit. Because this is similar to other patterns we've noticed and I hate that you're stuck in this web of self-judgment and self-criticism. Do you notice it and see how intense it seems? It makes me so sad. [responsive style—self-disclosure]

STEVE: Yeah, I mean, some of these are like more intense judgments then like "Oh, I'm not good at anything."

THERAPIST: That's where your mind goes. Did you have that thought on stage? Even as you were winning that award?

STEVE: Yeah, like I'm a big fraud.

THERAPIST: Oh, that sounds so so painful.

STEVE: Yeah, and I think it was worse because I also feel like I just didn't start my day right. I didn't even mention that my sleep has been totally messed up and I had like five cups of coffee that morning.

THERAPIST: So there were some major vulnerability factors too. Lack of sleep, lots of caffeine, definitely make you agitated, right?

STEVE: Yeah. I think the graduation would have been crummy anyway but the coffee probably didn't help.

THERAPIST: OK, so all this was going through your head while you're on the stage. You're like stuck in a thought tornado. [dialectical strategy: metaphor]

STEVE: Ha! That's a good one—"thought tornado"—it's totally true.

THERAPIST: Steve, let's finish up this chain. There's still a piece missing for me. How did you go from being on stage to in your car, burning yourself?

STEVE: As soon as my award was over, I went back toward my table at the back of the room. They had called up the next award winner to the stage so everyone was still focused on that. I was planning on sitting down, but I think I just sort of impulsively grabbed my stuff and left without saying goodbye to anyone.

THERAPIST: And you went straight to your car?

STEVE: Yeah. And I took out a cigarette and started smoking and then, barely thinking about it, I burned myself.

THERAPIST: Damn! *(loudly)* [irreverence]

STEVE: *(startled)* What?

THERAPIST: You missed a perfect opportunity to sit with all these negative feelings without escaping. [dialectical strategy: making lemonade out of lemons]

STEVE: It didn't feel so perfect at the time.

THERAPIST: Oh I get that completely. And let's be clear, by "perfect," I don't mean easy. I do think that learning how to tolerate difficult feelings will be a really important aspect of our treatment.

STEVE: Yeah, I know they're not going to go away completely.

THERAPIST: Just a few more questions. How long was it between when you got in your car and burned yourself with the cigarette?

STEVE: I don't know. It might have been less than a minute.

THERAPIST: And prior to getting in the car, were you aware of any urges to burn yourself?

STEVE: No, I think I was so caught up with what was happening, I didn't think of it at all until I was finally by myself.

THERAPIST: And so it was pretty impulsive? That moment of having an urge and then doing it? Doesn't sound like there was a lot of time in between.

STEVE: No, not at all.

THERAPIST: And did you have any thoughts at all about doing something different? About not injuring yourself?

STEVE: For a split second, I thought that you would be disappointed but then I put that out of my mind.

THERAPIST: Oh dear. You only thought of me for a nanosecond?! I think we're going to have to plaster pictures of me all over your car or your cigarette packs or something! [irreverence: unexpected response]

STEVE: Ha ha, that would be funny.

THERAPIST: Oh I'm being dead serious. *(pause)* OK, we have our work cut out for us, and I know we can do it. So now let's go back and figure out what you could have done differently so we can make sure burning never happens again. . . .

Commentary

In this fairly lengthy chain, the therapist has assessed the sequence of events leading up to the problem behavior of self-injury by burning, as well as some of the consequences. There were instances of validation, stylistic strategies, and dialectical strategies woven in, as needed. Their use was judicious and the therapist always kept her eye on the goal of completing a chain in order to more fully understand the behavior. Together, these strategies kept both the client and the therapist engaged and navigated potential landmines that would have otherwise derailed the chain. The therapist could use these strategies and keep focused on the process of the assessment.

In this chapter, I have reviewed a number of other strategies that are core features of DBT with an eye toward how they best can be used in the context of chain analyses. It is my hope that readers can see how the strategies are woven into chain analyses specifically. In fact, there is no natural separation between these strategies and chain analyses. Validation, reciprocal communication, irreverence, and dialectical strategies can all be used throughout chains to enhance their effectiveness.

CHAPTER 5

Incorporating Solutions into Chains

When a chain analysis is complete, one is left with an understanding of the factors that led to and followed a behavior one wants to change. A natural question is, "Now what?" The next task is to look for solutions that will lead to an increase in effective behavior and a decrease in the target behavior. A primary tenet of DBT and cognitive-behavioral treatments more generally is that awareness of causes of behavior, or "insight," is not sufficient. The client usually also needs to learn new strategies for changing the sequence of events in the future. To be clear, this book is not intended to review all of problem solving or the full scope of cognitive-behavioral solutions. However, it is impossible to fully teach how to competently conduct chain analyses without also delving into discussion of solutions. To that end, in this chapter, I provide a brief overview of the types of solutions offered in DBT and then focus on the process of incorporating solutions into chain analyses. More in-depth discussion of solutions can be found in Linehan (1993) and Heard and Swales (2015).

A Brief Overview of Solutions in DBT

I have found it helpful to always remind myself that the possible solutions in DBT fall into four categories: (1) skills training, (2) cognitive modification, (3) exposure, and (4) contingency management. Each of these categories influences different aspects of the chain analysis. The first three categories typically operate at the antecedent links of the chain (i.e., before the target behavior occurs). Contingency management operates at the consequences stage (after the target behavior occurs). See Figure 5.1.

This overview summarizes the solutions in each category to demonstrate the full range of possibilities. I will return to the chain of Steve's self-injury from the previous chapter to illustrate the possible solutions for him in each category but without settling on the *one or two* solutions that we might choose to implement. Generating ideas for possible solutions is only one step in learning how to incorporate solutions into chains.

Skills Training

When links in a chain are related to a skills deficit, then one solution is to teach the client the skills needed to overcome that deficit. The skills formally taught in DBT can be found in the DBT skills manual (Linehan, 2015). But it is important here to think about skills deficits more broadly and not necessarily linked to a particular skill. For example, if a link in the chain that led up to the client's avoidance behavior was related to him not knowing how to look for jobs effectively, a therapist may then teach the client the "skill" of job searching or connect him to someone who can help him in this area. If a link clearly highlighted the client's lack of skill in asking for something directly, the therapist may teach (or reteach) the client the interpersonal effectiveness skill of DEAR MAN for learning to get an objective (Linehan, 2015). DEAR MAN is an acronym for the steps of the skill: Describe (the situation), Express (your feelings and opinions), Assert (what you want), Reinforce (the person ahead of time), (be) Mindful, Appear confident, and (be willing to) Negotiate. Similarly, there are lots of times when a client demonstrates problem-solving skills deficits in a myriad of ways. Since DBT conceptualizes problems from a skills deficit model, there are usually multiple ways in which skills training could help change the chain of events in a more effective way.

For example, in the case of Steve's self-injury, we might ask what skills deficits were apparent during the chain of events. Related to specific DBT skills, we might notice that there was an absence of mindfulness (i.e., attention control) during the graduation ceremony. Instead of being present to the moment, he was "in his head" making comparisons and judgments. Similarly, there were skills deficits related to vulnerability factors that could be addressed by attending to the emotion regulation PLEASE skills. These are all focused on taking care of the mind by taking care of the body such as healthy eating, getting sufficient sleep, and

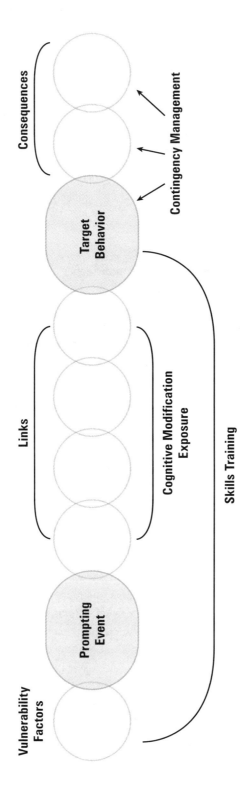

FIGURE 5.1. Chain analysis and DBT solution categories.

exercise. Specifically, Steve could reduce caffeine intake (the PLEASE skill of "avoid mood-altering substances"). This behavioral change would likely help reduce his vulnerability to extreme agitation. Then there are perhaps more subtle forms of skills deficit present in Steve's chain. At the end of the chain, the therapist labeled one without specifically using skills language by suggesting that Steve needs to learn how to sit with difficult feelings without escaping. This is an example of something that might not be typically thought of as a skill and yet is a strategy that a person can learn to do with practice (see also "Exposure" section below). The therapist could also tie it to the specific DBT skill of mindfulness of current emotions (Linehan, 2015).

Cognitive Modification

The solution set of cognitive modification refers to working directly with ineffective or maladaptive cognitions. These thoughts may show up on the chain either before or after the problem behavior. Notice that I use the words "ineffective" and "maladaptive" to describe the cognitions, rather than the words "faulty" or "distorted" that one often sees in the cognitive therapy literature. The reason for this choice of words is that, in the process of determining the controlling variables for a problematic behavior, cognitions that are a target in DBT may or may not be "accurate" or "true." An accurate thought may still cause problems. The focus on cognitions in chain analyses is more often about how particular thoughts contribute to the occurrence of the problem behavior rather than the *content* of the thought. For example, after failing a test at school, a client may think, "I suck at math," which leads down a path to his withdrawal in bed and failure to study for the next day. If the therapist focuses on the content of the thought, he or she might work hard with the client to get him to think that he doesn't "suck" at math. This is often a desire of therapists who don't like their clients having negative thoughts about themselves or their capabilities. However, to many clients, such restructuring can be perceived as invalidating and/or a "Pollyanna" approach to their problems. The "truth" is that they might not be gifted with math and they may never perform exceptionally well in math tests. Thus, in the context of chain analysis, the thought "I suck at math" might be identified as a critical variable in need of a solution, but the solution may be less about changing the content of the thought and more about figuring out what the thought does and how that function might be addressed or corrected in other more adaptive ways. In this case, the thought might be highlighted as a problematic link, and the therapist might work with the client to either come up with alternative thoughts or to incorporate more mindfulness into the moment ("The thought that I suck at math just went through my mind") in an effort to break the link between thought and behavior ("Therefore, I must withdraw from the world"). Cognitive modification as a set of solutions in DBT offers great flexibility.

> An ineffective thought might be identified as a critical variable, but the solution may be less about changing the content of the thought and more about understanding the function of the thought and how to address or correct that function in other more adaptive ways.

Steve appeared to have a number of cognitions in the lead-up to the self-injury that may have contributed to its occurrence. Some of these thoughts revolved around his relationship with Rachel, which he thought was "fake"; he also thought that others at the graduation ceremony were judging him. Closer in time to the self-injury, he had thoughts that he wasn't good at anything. From within the solution category of cognitive modification, the therapist has a number of options available. The therapist could work with Steve to directly modify those thoughts, such as from thinking "I'm not good at anything" to something more realistic like "There are some things (specify) that I excel at." A DBT therapist might also directly challenge or confront problematic thoughts using irreverent styles as discussed in the previous chapter, in order to highlight the ways in which the thoughts cause problems for Steve and get him to think differently about the situation. In addition, the therapist might help Steve to observe and describe his thoughts and their effects on his behavior and emotions. For example, "So you had the thought that you weren't good at anything. Did you notice that as just a thought? How can we get you to approach your thoughts this way instead of as facts?" In this way, the therapist is incorporating the "mindfulness of thoughts" skill that teaches how to experience thoughts without necessarily acting on them. Finally, the therapist might incorporate other strategies for reducing the likelihood that these thoughts affect his behavior, for example, noticing the "thought tornado" as it was occurring and distracting from it or using it as a cue to engage in more active behavior.

Exposure

The solution of exposure involves working directly with conditioned responses between stimuli and emotional responses that lead to the problem behavior. In my experience, exposure is the category of solutions least likely to be thought of and implemented by the therapist. Therapists may have a knowledge deficit, having never been taught how to look for classically conditioned emotional responses nor how to use exposure to break these conditioned associations. Or, therapists may avoid exposure due to their own discomfort with causing their client intense negative emotion through exposure procedures. However, if a therapist is not considering exposure as a solution, he or she is likely missing opportunities to solve the problem effectively.

Although formal use of exposure in the form of protocols may be warranted in the systematic treatment of particular problems like PTSD (posttraumatic stress disorder), DBT frequently favors the use of informal exposure when relevant in particular chains of behavior. That is, when a problematic link on the chain involves a conditioned emotional response, the therapist can work to directly intervene at that link without incorporating a more formal protocol. Conditioned emotional responses frequently take the form of *avoidance behavior*. For example, the client who failed a math test [prompting event], had the thought "I suck at math" [link: thought], felt intense shame and anxiety [link: emotion], and then withdrew to bed for the rest of the day and slept [problem behavior] to escape the negative feelings he experienced [consequence]. Exposure would likely be an effective solution here. The therapist might assess the client's degree of shame over failing the exam to be out of proportion to the event itself. Thus, an exposure could involve having the client keep talking in session about failing the exam in a more matter-of-fact manner as a means to decrease the experience of shame in relation to the event. By doing so, the client also learns that he can tolerate the shame without having to resort to ineffective behaviors. The idea here is that intense shame is causing problems for the client, and thus reducing shame (via exposure to the event that elicits it) would help the client engage in more adaptive behavior subsequently.

Steve experienced intense emotions of shame and anger that he avoided by engaging in self-injury. Exposure as a solution could involve intentionally eliciting those same emotions in session and having Steve "ride them out" without engaging in problematic behavior. The point of this exercise, which would likely need to be repeated several times within or between sessions, would be for Steve to learn that emotions will lessen over time on their own *and* that he can tolerate them. In so doing, the link between the antecendent and the behavior becomes broken and new links are forged.

Contingency Management

In contrast to the other solution sets, contingency management focuses on events in a chain that occur *after* the problem behavior. Specifically, contingency management involves changing a target behavior's consequences, such that it is less likely to be reinforced (or more likely to be punished) and that effective alternative behavior is more likely to be reinforced. Solutions might involve adding in specific reinforcers for adaptive behavior, like rewarding oneself or involving a friend or family member to help in providing reinforcement. The relevant solution might also focus on shaping the client's environment so that it responds more effectively to target behaviors. Contingency management might also involve adding a negative consequence to the behavior one is trying to decrease. The 24-hour rule in DBT is one such negative consequence, in that a client is not allowed to reach out to his or her therapist for any unscheduled calls in the 24 hours following a self-injury. The absence of therapist availability following a self-injurious act is intended to function as an aversive consequence that a client might naturally want to avoid (thus reducing the likelihood of self-injury in the future).

In Steve's case, a clear contingency was the immediate relief he felt after burning himself. This experience is common with self-injury and substance use; the immediate consequences are quite powerful and difficult to directly change. Even though he said he very quickly returned to feeling "crummy," the bad news about contingencies is that this immediate relief is likely more powerful for maintaining the behavior than the subsequent guilt and shame. Thus, the therapist might have to be creative in solution generation for contingencies. Focusing on immediate reinforcement of alternative skillful behaviors is critical, as is thinking of ways to add in aversives for the self-injury. For Steve, this might mean working on having him reach out to the therapist prior to self-injury as an alternative and then reinforcing this behavior with praise, validation, and help. It might also mean determining an aversive contingency to add immediately following a self-injury to counteract the positive physiological response. For example, the therapist can have Steve complete a chain analysis on his own self-injury *as soon as possible* after the self-injury. As discussed previously, while chain analysis itself is not intended to be punishment, we could hypothesize that this would not be a preferred activity immediately after the behavior. Thus, adding it as close as possible to the behavior may serve to punish the behavior. Steve might think twice before engaging in self-injury if he knew he would have to perform a task immediately after it.

As you can see, these four categories cover a lot of terrain when it comes to possible solutions. The reason I find it helpful to remember these broad categories, rather than specific solutions, is that it reminds the therapist of the myriad of opportunities that are available, rather than get stuck on one solution (e.g., skills training) that may have only limited effectiveness for the particular problem because it doesn't address a critical link. Each of these solution sets essentially addresses different links in the chain. Keeping the solutions in mind can help the therapist generate specific questions for him- or herself and the client. The questions in Table 5.1 can guide the assessment.

Of course, in many circumstances, all four of these questions are answered yes. This leads to the next topic: determining what solutions might be the best ones to go for during the chain analysis.

Determining the "Best" Solution to Implement

Now that all the possibilities for solutions have been reviewed, it is easy to see how a therapist and client might be overwhelmed with the sheer

TABLE 5.1. Questions for Identifying Solutions

Is there a notable skills deficit?	Solution: Skills training
Are there ineffective cognitions?	Solution: Cognitive modification
Are intense emotions interfering?	Solution: Exposure
Are there problematic contingencies?	Solution: Contingency management

number of alternatives. Indeed, if every link in the chain is associated with at least one possible alternative, one could easily identify 20–30 "solutions" for each chain. However, *not all links are created equal*. It is important for the therapist to keep two priorities in mind when choosing solutions that the client is asked to implement. One priority is finding a solution that addresses a critical variable in the chain such that, if this solution is implemented, you have the greatest chance of changing the target behavior in a lasting way. The second priority is finding a solution that can be easily implemented and has a chance of changing the target behavior at least for the short term. Although the first priority reflects the ultimate goal of addressing the target behavior, it can often take time to address and be difficult to implement. Thus, focus on "easy" solutions to prevent the target behavior while working on the longer-term items. For example, a client's chronic and global insomnia could be a critical link (vulnerability factor) in subsequent substance use. While strategies for addressing insomnia will ultimately prove extremely successful in reducing substance use, it will take weeks to implement. Thus, in the short term, the therapist might also teach some short-term distress tolerance strategies to address a later link that also contributes to substance use.

> Keep two priorities in mind when choosing a solution: (1) find a solution that targets a variable with the greatest chance of enduring change and (2) find a solution that can be easily implemented.

Note that it is not helpful to pick a solution that would have only worked in that one particular instance if that instance is unlikely to occur again. There may have been a perfect solution for that one particular instance of behavior but that solution doesn't translate well to other circumstances in which risk of the target behavior is high. Imagine an adolescent client who engaged in drinking behavior (target behavior) during senior prom (a once-in-a-lifetime event). The therapist would want to look for links in the chain that are more relevant to drinking behavior in general (e.g., feelings of hurt that arise in interpersonal situations, peer pressure) or related to a multitude of other target behaviors (e.g., seeking to escape the experience of shame) and focus less on links that are solely related to prom even if they affected the subsequent drinking (e.g., her prom date was late picking her up; something spilled on her new dress during dinner). Focusing on the latter would likely lead to a discussion of "how could prom have gone differently" which may not be at all helpful now that prom is a thing of the past! Instead, the focus should be on "how can we get you to not drink again" and thus focusing on the links that are more relevant across broader contexts and situations.

Regardless of which solutions are chosen to implement, it is extremely important to look for ways in which that solution could be immediately taught or practiced in session. It is often not helpful for the therapist to say, "OK, so we've determined that doing DEAR MANs would be helpful for you so go and practice this week." If clients knew how to successfully integrate skillful behavior in their lives, they would be doing so already! Thus, the therapist has to leave time in session to plan for how the solutions will be incorporated, practice in session if at all possible, and troubleshoot any problems that might arise in the practice and application. Ideally, a new solution or behavior is practiced in every session.

Weaving Solutions into Chains versus Waiting Until the Chain Is Complete

The most commonly asked question about incorporating solutions into chain analyses is *When?* Is it preferable to weave in solutions as one notices problematic links or is it better to wait until the chain is complete and then go back to incorporate solutions? The answer is ultimately the unsatisfying "It depends." There are pros and cons for each method, which I'll detail below and in Table 5.2.

I advise novice DBT clinicians to work first on getting the complete chain before shifting to solutions. The primary reason for this is that if you focus on a specific solution too early in the chain, you may miss the most relevant aspect that comes later. More experienced clinicians may find that weaving solutions in as they go offers opportunities to directly impact relevant links as they arise. A middle path is to highlight places where solutions will be incorporated as you conduct the chain without specifically doing the solution analysis yet. For example, a therapist might say, "It seems like this moment when you had the thought 'I suck at math' may have really set you up; I have lots of ideas for how we might address that, so let's remember to come back to this."

TABLE 5.2. Pros and Cons of When to Incorporate Solutions in Chain Analyses

Weaving in solutions as you go	Completing the entire chain first
Pros	Pros
• Can strike while the iron is hot by working on a problematic link when talking about it. • Can be more hope generating for client since possible solutions are identified and implemented right away.	• Can get the entire picture of the chain, which will prevent premature rushing to solutions without full assessment. • More likely to identify the critical links. • Allows client to tell the "whole story" with minimal interruption.
Cons	Cons
• May run out of session time without completing full chain. • May miss the critical link by focusing too soon on other solutions.	• May run out of session time without spending adequate time on solutions, leading to potential hopelessness and/or lack of change.

Illustration of Incorporation of Solutions after the Chain Is Complete

I'll return to where the therapist left off with Steve in the last chapter. In broad strokes, the completed chain looks like Figure 5.2. Options for some possible solutions have been highlighted above in each of the solution categories sections and here I present a transcript of the discussion between Steve and his therapist following the chain. Remember that the therapist is working with Steve to identify two things: (1) where solutions might be easy to implement and (2) what solutions might be most critical to changing the problem behavior over the long term. For illustration purposes, I'm working under the assumption that Steve is committed to reducing his self-injury behavior and thus commitment does not need to be addressed here.

THERAPIST: So now let's go back and figure out what you could have done differently so we can make sure burning never happens again. (*Refers to written-out visual of chain.*) The good news is that it looks to me like there were a lot of opportunities to get things to go a

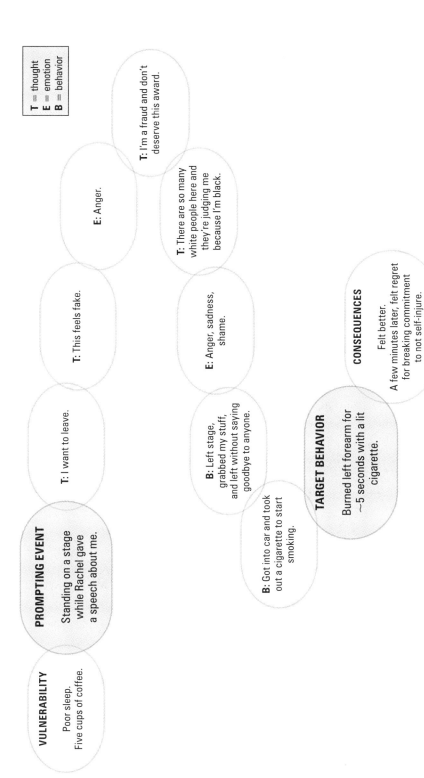

VULNERABILITY

Poor sleep.
Five cups of coffee.

PROMPTING EVENT

Standing on a stage while Rachel gave a speech about me.

T: I want to leave.

T: This feels fake.

E: Anger.

T: I'm a fraud and don't deserve this award.

T: There are so many white people here and they're judging me because I'm black.

E: Anger, sadness, shame.

B: Left stage, grabbed my stuff, and left without saying goodbye to anyone.

B: Got into car and took out a cigarette to start smoking.

TARGET BEHAVIOR

Burned left forearm for ~5 seconds with a lit cigarette.

CONSEQUENCES

Felt better.
A few minutes later, felt regret for breaking commitment to not self-injure.

T = thought
E = emotion
B = behavior

FIGURE 5.2. Chain analysis of Steve's burning behavior.

107

different way. That doesn't mean it's easy, it just means that we have a lot to work with.

STEVE: Yeah, OK.

THERAPIST: I have my own ideas but I also want to ask you: what do you think is the most critical link here? Meaning, if this one link didn't happen, the self-injury wouldn't have happened.

STEVE: Hmm. Probably having to go to the graduation.

THERAPIST: Ah, yeah, that might be true. That if you didn't have the prompting event of the graduation ceremony, you wouldn't have self-injured. So, one option would be to just avoid all events that might prompt emotions of any kind. [irreverence: joking, light tone] And that is a solution but probably not one that fits with your goals and values. So what other link seems critical to you?

STEVE: A couple of things I guess. One is that all the coffee and stuff made me really jittery and I think if I wasn't as agitated at the ceremony, things would have gone differently.

THERAPIST: OK, that's really helpful to know. If you weren't as agitated, you might not have experienced the thought tornado?

STEVE: Not as bad.

THERAPIST: Very useful. OK, what was the other thing?

STEVE: I think as soon as I got in my car feeling the way I felt, I was doomed.

THERAPIST: Yes! I think the same thing. To me, leaving the ceremony to go be by yourself in the car when you were feeling such intense emotions was a major red flag. Just to be clear, do you think if you went to have a cigarette outside but not in your car, you would have burned yourself?

STEVE: No, I don't think so. I would have been worried that someone would see me.

THERAPIST: So being in your car where people couldn't see you was critical. And being alone with very intense emotions.

STEVE: Yes.

THERAPIST: OK we have a lot to work with, this is good! I also want to put out there that some of the thoughts that you were having about race and otherness seem really important to address because they cause a lot of suffering even if they don't always lead to self-injury. I'd like us to return to that after we get your self-harm under control because I think it would be helpful—what about you?

STEVE: Yeah, I do want to talk about that. I feel like I have so much I want to get off my chest always.

THERAPIST: Good, we are on the same page. Let's get self-injury out of your life so we can turn to these bigger issues. So there are two things that I think we can do to address self-injury risk this week. One is I'm wondering if we could reduce your agitation by limiting your caffeine intake, no matter how bad your sleep was the night before.

STEVE: Yeah, I think that's a good idea.

THERAPIST: What is a reasonable amount to you? Two cups? Would that make you as agitated?

STEVE: I can try two. It might be difficult when I'm really tired though.

THERAPIST: Well, what if we just did an experiment for a couple of weeks? No more than two cups of coffee a day and we can add a couple of columns to your diary card for caffeine intake and degree of agitation? And if it doesn't have much of an impact, we can reevaluate?

STEVE: Yeah, I like that idea.

THERAPIST: Great. (*Adds columns to diary card.*) The second thing might be harder and so I also want to look for ways for us to practice it in session. It has to do with feeling intense emotions without immediately engaging in some impulsive behavior that you later regret.

STEVE: That's definitely an issue for me.

THERAPIST: I know. And I get it. Most people have difficulty tolerating really intense negative emotions and do many things to try to avoid the experience. Ultimately, though, when we avoid, we never learn that feelings are just feelings, they may be uncomfortable and unpleasant but they're not going to hurt us and they will eventually dissipate. Do you see that?

STEVE: Logically, I get that. But in the moment, it's really hard. I just want to escape immediately.

THERAPIST: Right. And it takes lots of practice. Perhaps more so for you because you've built up such a strong habit of escape. So the trick here is mindfulness and specifically mindfulness of emotions. I know you've learned this in group and we need to integrate it more into your life. [Note: mindfulness of emotion is both a skill and an exposure exercise.] You remember what it is?

STEVE: Yeah, it's just observing your experience.

THERAPIST: Exactly! Observing your emotions with some distance and just allowing them to do what they do without acting on any of the urges to arise. Can we practice that?

STEVE: Sure.

Here the therapist would work with Steve to generate some negative emotions in session, likely by going back to the links in the chain that were particularly evocative. Then she would lead Steve through a mindfulness of emotion exercise in order to practice and also so the therapist can observe any obstacles or misapplications and address them in the moment. Before ending the session, she would work to get a commitment from Steve to practice mindfulness of emotions a certain number of times, or in certain situations, in the subsequent week while also offering phone coaching to help with its implementation.

Thus, after a chain is complete, the process of incorporating solutions embodies all the principles discussed in the previous chapters. It assumes that there is sufficient time in the session to both identify the one or two solutions the therapist wishes to implement and time to practice them. If there is not sufficient time, some of these discussions may carry over to the subsequent session or several sessions.

Illustration of Weaving Solutions into the Chain

In this illustration, I show how solutions can be woven into the chain as it's occurring. John was a 34-year-old man whose primary target behavior for treatment was binge eating. Despite an early commitment to not binge eat for the duration of treatment, he engaged in an episode approximately 2 months into treatment while he was away on vacation with his family of origin. Thus, this chain represents the first time an assessment was conducted on a binge-eating episode. In this chain, we see many of the elements of the previous chapters illustrated. However, we also see the incorporation of solutions within the chain, as well as an end to the chain that highlights what work will need to be explored in order to effectively change the target behavior over the long-term.

THERAPIST: Oh no, so the binge eating happened right after our phone conversation . . . what happened, how did you end up doing this?

JOHN: I went to the kitchen, grabbed a couple of things, and then went to my room and shoveled it all in. I've never done it someplace other than my own house before.

THERAPIST: Can you describe to me what you ate? [assessing target behavior]

JOHN: Ugh, I hate saying it out loud. Probably half a bag of Oreos and a container of chocolate ice cream.

THERAPIST: What size container?

JOHN: A half-gallon. Some of it was already eaten but most of it was still there.

THERAPIST: OK. And when did the thought first come up that you wanted to binge?

JOHN: I'm not sure . . . I got off the phone with you, it was probably about 20 minutes between when I talked to you and when it happened. I was feeling really bad, and I texted my wife about what I talked to you about. She was trying to help me. I didn't feel like I could do all of the steps that you and I talked about. I just wanted to go to bed instead of doing those steps. So I sort of wandered into the kitchen because I was hungry. It was in the kitchen that the frustration became really intense and I just all of a sudden grabbed those things.

THERAPIST: So you were feeling a lot of frustration just prior to binge eating. Just curious, what else do you think would have helped you get your frustration down then?

JOHN: I probably could have left the house, gotten some fresh air, and been away from my family.

THERAPIST: Would that have helped reduce the likelihood of bingeing?

JOHN: Yeah, I think so.

THERAPIST: OK, that's good to know. [Note that this generated solution was specific to some unique aspects of this chain: being on vacation with his family. Thus, the therapist is not going to spend too much time elaborating on this right now.] So you're in the kitchen, feeling frustrated. Tell me more about that moment.

JOHN: I was overthinking and getting really frustrated about the things we talked about. Like, ruminating.

THERAPIST: So frustrated on a level of?

JOHN: 5 [out of 5].

THERAPIST: And who or what were you frustrated with?

JOHN: My aunt.

THERAPIST: OK. So what had happened with your aunt?

JOHN: It was a cluster of things that happened . . . the day before my sister was crying and was really upset because my aunt was working all day even during parts of the day when we all were supposed to go out together sight-seeing.

THERAPIST: And your sister was upset about that?

JOHN: Yeah. And then there's always drama with my sister and mom and my aunt in general. So I was really upset that my sister was upset, on top of all of the normal stuff. And my younger sister is depressed right now, and we're all afraid that my younger sister is going to start self-harming. And we were talking about that too.

THERAPIST: Wow, so you had a ton of stuff going on, and a lot was on your mind. All of this happened the night and day before?

JOHN: Yeah.

THERAPIST: So that's some high emotional vulnerability factors, starting this day in a bad place, thinking about all this stuff from the night before. It seems like there were some huge warning signs going up that this was going to be a difficult day for you, right?

JOHN: Yeah. I didn't know I was going to binge but I knew it was going be a rough day.

THERAPIST: OK, so given all these warning signs, is there anything you could have done to reduce your vulnerability to engage in problematic behaviors? What could you have done when you first recognized this was going to be a difficult day? [targeting vulnerability factors]

JOHN: I probably could have worked out when I woke up.

THERAPIST: That sounds like a great idea! What would that have looked like specifically?

JOHN: I could have done some cardio—I had bought all my exercise clothes with me and there was a machine there. I just kept putting it off.

THERAPIST: OK, so exercising first thing in the morning sounds like a potentially good solution. I know exercising regularly is important to you and also we know that it reduces your vulnerability to negative emotions. Remember those PLEASE skills? *(John nods.)* Let's hold onto this idea. Did anything else happen this day?

JOHN: Yeah, so we were all feeling on edge I think. It was just a fiasco when my aunt finally got off the phone. We went somewhere for lunch, it was a really long wait, so we went somewhere else to eat but we couldn't find anything that was vegan, and it was annoying my aunt that my sister was vegan, and everyone was fighting in the car the whole way between lunch places about what we're doing.

THERAPIST: So a lot of high emotion and conflict with your family all afternoon.

JOHN: Yeah, and then we got into a conversation about my other aunt while in the car. She had said something hurtful to my sister the other week, and we were complaining about it, and this aunt defended her, saying, "Oh well, she probably didn't mean to" and defending her and not being on our side about it, and my sister was getting really upset, and I couldn't help but get really upset too because she was upset.

THERAPIST: How were you feeling then?

JOHN: I was really mad in the car.

THERAPIST: Anger?

JOHN: Definitely. At a 5 [out of 5]. At my aunt. And my aunt had teased me about wanting to get more food, making jokes about me eating.

THERAPIST: Oh no . . .

JOHN: Yeah, and I hadn't gone to the gym this week so it just really sucked to have to think about that. And then she ditched us when we got to the mall, which was so lame, because she just wanted to go shopping and at that point I'm just like "I'm done with this" and . . .

THERAPIST: Can you bring us back to here? *(pointing at a link in the chain)* So, you had a lot of family conflict earlier in the day, for sure. And now you're in the car feeling really angry. What could you have done right then? Something to either reduce your anger right away or help you tolerate it better so that it's less likely to lead to you bingeing? [another solution discussion, keeping in mind the goal of trying to prevent the target behavior]

JOHN: I could feel myself getting worked up in the car but I was also sort of trapped in there. So maybe some of that distraction skill would have helped—like counting up to a certain number or something.

THERAPIST: Oh, that's a really great one! I'm so proud of you for generating that idea right now. That's exactly the sort of mental skill that can help in situations where escape is difficult. [skill as solution: distraction from the distress tolerance module] I like to take a moment and just focus on my breath for 10 deep breaths because you can do that anywhere. Would that have been an option?

JOHN: Yeah, that would have been good too. And maybe even more helpful.

THERAPIST: OK, let's keep this in mind too. So what was happening later at night? What was happening right before you called me?

JOHN: I got workout stuff together, trying to be good. "OK, I'm gonna work out and do cardio." I got to the machine and I realized I had to take my shoes off again to stretch and I thought "I just can't do this."

THERAPIST: Exercise?

JOHN: Yeah. Just like something was immediately thrown away and I couldn't get myself back on the machine.

THERAPIST: How were you feeling? I know overwhelmed; any specific emotions?

JOHN: I guess it's kind of like anger . . .

THERAPIST: Anger at what?

JOHN: Like, my aunt, but also the cosmos. Like, one more thing is being thrown at me, it's not fair, and I just can't stand it, like what's the point of doing anything. So like, anger at a level of 5. And I was still angry at my aunt a lot too, for not even caring that she was upsetting my sister. I was just so over her and over everything.

THERAPIST: Ugh, uh huh. So it sounds like a lot of "should" statements showed up—your aunt should be different, the world should be different, right?

JOHN: Exactly.

THERAPIST: Those thoughts get you in trouble! We've talked about these thoughts before, how they really lead you down the path of pretty ineffective behavior, as they would do for anyone if you start thinking them enough. Let's just take a quick moment to think about this—going back to that moment, anything you could have done differently when you had that first "should" thought? [solutions: cognitive modification]

JOHN: Well, I guess the first thing would be noticing I'm having them.

THERAPIST: Yes! Exactly! So observing your thoughts might be very important. If you had said to yourself "Oh, those thoughts about how things should be different are showing up," what might you have done differently?

JOHN: Hmm, not sure. I think I was so angry, I'm not sure it would have made much difference.

THERAPIST: OK, so let's put that one aside for now. It's possible that when your emotions are at a certain intensity, it's hard for you to think differently. This is true for loads of people, including me. And I think it's important for us to figure out, in the long run, how to reduce some of these thoughts because they definitely contribute. Do you agree?

JOHN: Yes, totally.

THERAPIST: So after got off the phone with me, what did you do?

JOHN: I texted Amy [wife] because she had told me that I should call you. And I told her it was too late to call you, and she said she didn't think that was true so I agreed to try to call you . . .

THERAPIST: That was awesome.

JOHN: . . . and so I was texting her to tell her that I talked to you. And then I made the mistake of rehashing everything with my family with her.

THERAPIST: Ah. And you're saying now that that was a mistake. What makes you say that?

JOHN: Well, I had been feeling better after I talked with you and then I got all riled up again.

THERAPIST: I see that entirely. So after you got off the phone with me, what could you have done differently?

JOHN: I could have texted Amy that we talked and then not said more about my family stuff.

THERAPIST: OK, that's something you could have *not* done. What behavior could you have done instead?

JOHN: I could have gone straight into the shower like you and I had talked about.

THERAPIST: Right. You and I had talked more generally about doing something to distract yourself in a positive way. What else could you have done right then?

JOHN: We talked about me looking for comedy videos.

THERAPIST: Right. Would that have helped?

JOHN: Yeah, probably. But I got caught up with the texting instead.

THERAPIST: Hmm, OK, we're going to have to return to troubleshooting what gets in the way of you engaging in skillful behavior when you know that it will likely help. Anyway, for now, let's go back to you and Amy texting.

JOHN: I texted her that I just talked to you, and that you helped me with anger, and that I was really mad, and here's why I'm really mad . . . and then I got really really mad telling her about why I was mad *(laughing)*. Ugh and I knew it, and I even told her "I can't talk about this or I'm not supposed to talk about this, because I'm supposed to be distracting myself."

THERAPIST: Mm-hmm. So you definitely didn't do our plan! I totally get why it would be hard not to talk to your wife about the thing upsetting you, and at the same time that's what we're seeing as being really important for you . . . to not ruminate when you're feeling that upset, because we know that gets you really overwhelmed by things.

JOHN: Yeah. But my feeling at that point was I don't care about being effective and not ruminating, I just don't care.

THERAPIST: OK, so some willfulness showed up.

JOHN: Yeah, I guess so.

THERAPIST: Yeah, that's what your anger at the cosmos sounds like. Ugh, stamping your feet at reality and then not wanting to do anything about it.

JOHN: Yeah.

THERAPIST: And then that ended up making things worse in the long run.

JOHN: Yeah, that's definitely true.

THERAPIST: Anything you could have done there to reduce your willfulness? What about willing hands or half-smile, or both? [DBT skill aimed at decreasing willfulness and increasing acceptance using one's body]

JOHN: That didn't even occur to me.

THERAPIST: Exactly! We need to get these options to show up in your mind. Instead you ended up binge eating. And what happened here (*pointing at "binge" on the written chain*), when you ate those Oreos and ice cream?

JOHN: It totally helped.

THERAPIST: It worked, like your anger went down to 0?

JOHN: Is this in the actual moment or right after?

THERAPIST: That's a great distinction—you tell me.

JOHN: In the moment there was no anger, like 0. I felt totally numbed out. And then right after, I had maybe a 2 or 3 of anger. Because I knew my aunt was downstairs ignoring the whole thing.

THERAPIST: Any other emotions pop up?

JOHN: I had a lot of shame because I knew I had done that. Like a level of 4. And I was still feeling willful. And I didn't want to call you any more because I'd binged and was feeling disgusted and embarrassed about that.

THERAPIST: Oh, so that's why you didn't text me like we'd planned. Yeah, I was bummed by that.

JOHN: Yeah, I know . . .

THERAPIST: OK. So back during your conversation with your wife before the binge . . . can you tell me a little bit about that?

JOHN: She was coaching me, a little bit like you would, but I mostly ignored her. She also was trying to comfort me and make me feel better, but she was more trying to push me. I was just sitting on the floor texting her the whole time until I decided to get up to go to the kitchen.

THERAPIST: So when you went into the kitchen, were you intending to binge?

JOHN: No. Didn't even think about it.

THERAPIST: And then—

JOHN: I was still just turning over everything in my head. Because when I had come into the kitchen, I passed by everyone in the living room and it made me think about it all over again. Thinking about the car conversation the day before where she wasn't calling the other aunt out.

THERAPIST: About the car conversation?!

JOHN: Ugh, I know, I know.

THERAPIST: OK. So. What do you see in this chain? I've highlighted some things and we've already talked about a lot of possible solutions, but I want to hear what you learn from looking at everything like this.

JOHN: So . . . I think I learned that I can be mindful because I told my wife that I'm going to vent when I shouldn't *(laughing)*.

THERAPIST: OK! So you were mindful of your willfulness.

JOHN: Yeah, I didn't call it that then, but I did notice it.

THERAPIST: OK! And that's a pretty big deal for you. The first step in addressing willfulness is noticing it. That's not easy to do. In the past you've gotten in trouble for getting into rumination without realizing it, and you don't even have a chance to practice a skill, and it makes it really worse really quickly for you. So at least noticing it here is a big deal. We're going to practice willing hands in a minute.

JOHN: OK.

THERAPIST: OK. . . . What else do you notice?

JOHN: I think . . . the self-validating thing.

THERAPIST: Oh?

JOHN: Yeah, it's just a lot of sucky crap.

THERAPIST: Yeah! This does not sound like a very fun vacation day!

JOHN: But that's not something I noticed until the whole week was over, so I think the self-validation thing could've helped during it.

THERAPIST: Of course. OK. Let's go back through everything, and talk about times you could've self-validated, self-soothed, and practiced the other skills to help you get through these tough times.

This chain with John is an example of how more discussion of solutions can be incorporated into the chain as the chain is occurring, rather than waiting until every detail has been obtained. As highlighted, there were many potential points of intervention and the therapist "struck while the iron was hot" by asking John what he could have done differently at the moments they were discussing. This often helps the client see it more readily in his mind's eye and may be more likely to accurately assess whether the offered solution is feasible or likely to work. The solutions covered included skills training and cognitive modification. The therapist might make note of the fact that she only covered these two solution categories and subsequently might see whether using exposure or contingency management would be useful.

It is important to keep the ultimate goal of chain analyses in mind: you are working to increase effective behaviors and decrease ineffective behaviors. This can yield more helpful questions during the chain that move you toward effective and practical solutions. More specifically, the therapist needs to recognize that the chain analysis is not just information for information's sake. In this chapter, I discussed the different solutions and areas of the chain that they are meant to address. There are a lot of choice points in solution implementation: Which links in the chain to target? Which solutions are "best" in preventing the behavior from occurring again in the future? When is the best time to discuss solutions, during the chain or after? While there is no one right answer to these questions, knowing the possibilities affords the therapist flexibility.

However, even when solutions are generated in the context of the chain, they don't always work. One aspect of working with clients with a long history of problem behaviors is that these behaviors have been excessively rehearsed and are frequently habitual. It takes effort and stamina to counteract these long histories and generate new habits in the form of more effective behaviors.

In the next chapter, I address some of these issues by discussing the process of conducting repeated chains on the same behavior—that is, what to do when a behavior continues to occur even after completing one or more chain analyses.

CHAPTER 6

When a Behavior Isn't Changing

There is a widely held misconception that an "assessment phase" occurs in early sessions and then is completed prior to turning toward a "treatment phase." However, the stance in behavioral treatments is that assessment never ends. In fact, it is impossible to separate assessment and treatment because they are so critically interwoven. For example, assessment happens in every session that a client did not do an assigned task ("What got in the way of completing the task?"; "Did you think about doing it when you left the session?"; etc.). Assessment happens every time a new problem behavior shows up, assessment happens every time a problem behavior fails to change despite a proposed solution, and assessment can even happen when a new, functional behavior arises that the therapist wants to strengthen. Indeed, if the behavior does not change, then there is likely to be an assessment error or deficiency. Assessment continues so that key themes across chains emerge and help the therapist effectively zero-in on the most critical factors influencing the target behaviors.

Of course, sometimes you "nail" a chain analysis the first time you do one. It becomes evident what the key controlling variable is; you address it with a solution that is easy to identify and implement; and the problem is solved. Voilà! However, it is usually the case that once is not enough and that the therapist will need to conduct multiple chains about the same behavior. The focus of this chapter is on how to continue to assess a behavior for which you have already conducted more than one chain. If a behavior has been previously assessed, solutions generated, and yet the behavior continues to occur, the question the therapist needs to ask is "What did I miss?" That is, the therapist needs to turn a critical eye toward understanding why the target behavior is not changing. A therapist may need to zoom in on a 1-minute section of the chain or zoom out and look to bigger-picture items that maintain the behavior.

The conduct of chain analyses inevitably changes over time. As the therapist gets to know the client and his or her patterns better, there may be less time spent on assessment of each individual link and more "short-cuts" may be taken to understand the sequence of events. The therapist may focus on a particular segment of the chain that is more poorly understood and/or most intransigent to solutions and not spend time on other pieces of the chain that have been shown to be less useful or relevant for solution generation.

For example, if a client was late to session by 15 minutes for the fourth time in 2 months, a therapist may conduct a "chain of lateness," but will already likely have a lot of information from the previous three occurrences. Rather than conduct the chain from scratch by asking detailed questions about events, thoughts, feelings, behaviors, and the like, he or she may instead have the following interaction:

THERAPIST: We need to talk about you being late to session by 15 minutes today. Let's do a chain of what happened and also figure out what got in the way of you trying the solutions we discussed the last time. When did you first know that you were going to be late?

CLIENT: When I finally woke up. I guess I pressed my snooze button about six times and when I finally woke up, it was an hour later than I was planning.

THERAPIST: What time was it that you set the alarm for and what time did you wake up?

CLIENT: I set it for 9:00. I didn't get out of bed until 10:15.

[The session was scheduled for 11:00, and the therapist is already aware that it takes the client 15 minutes to drive to the office.]

THERAPIST: OK, so a major problem is the multiple snoozes. We've talked about that before. I'm also wondering what time you went to bed last night?

CLIENT: I had a hard time falling asleep. I was probably up until about 4:00.

THERAPIST: Wow! OK. That would likely make it hard for anyone to wake up at 9:00, just 5 hours later. So not getting to sleep until that time likely made you very vulnerable to not waking up when your alarm first went off. Sleep dysregulation has come up a lot for you and we may have to spend some more time addressing that since it seems to be related to so many problems for you.

At this point, approximately 2 minutes have been spent discussing the target behavior of lateness. Unlike many of the chains illustrated in previous chapters, this one appears a bit different on the surface. However, the therapist is keeping the structure of the chain in her mind as she assesses and likely has an outline of the chain of events in her mind. It would look something like Figure 6.1.

If this was a first chain conducted on the client's lateness behavior, we would say it is insufficient in many ways. Links are assumed rather than assessed, and many pieces are missing. There is no focus on emotions or cognitions. However, this is a repeated chain done on the target of lateness, and therefore the therapist has some additional choice points. The therapist could take the time to flesh out all the unknown links or explore further the thoughts and emotions that go along with various steps of this specific chain. However, she has already completed a couple of chains on this behavior in previous sessions and has learned via those chains that, although emotions and thoughts are present in the sequence of events, they do not appear critically related to the target behavior of lateness. The therapist has also learned that knowing more about the intermediate links (e.g., between getting out of bed at 10:15 and leaving for the appointment at 11:00) will not yield a lot of helpful information regarding changing the problem. Therefore, she takes a shortcut and jumps over a piece of the chain that is likely irrelevant, based on her experience with previous chains. She zeroes in on the idea that not getting out of bed until 45 minutes before the session was scheduled to start was the primary controlling variable this time and in other instances previously assessed, and she suggests a solution (i.e., a series of steps for improving sleep hygiene) for this problem.

This illustration shows chain analyses can be much shorter in later sessions when multiple chains have already been completed. I want to emphasis this particular point because oftentimes clinicians believe that a chain analysis *must* include every minute detail from moment to moment. In so doing, they risk alienating their clients, who find this exercise tedious and ultimately unhelpful when it's repeated ad nauseum without any alterations depending on what number chain it is. It also

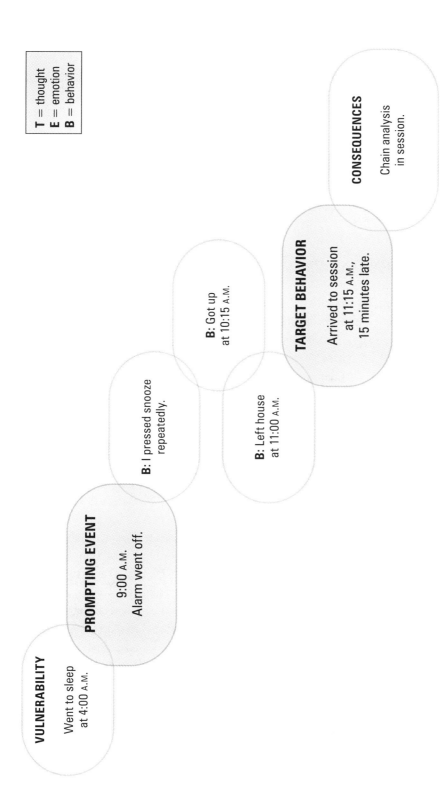

T = thought
E = emotion
B = behavior

VULNERABILITY

Went to sleep
at 4:00 A.M.

PROMPTING EVENT

9:00 A.M.
Alarm went off.

B: I pressed snooze
repeatedly.

B: Got up
at 10:15 A.M.

B: Left house
at 11:00 A.M.

TARGET BEHAVIOR

Arrived to session
at 11:15 A.M.,
15 minutes late.

CONSEQUENCES

Chain analysis
in session.

FIGURE 6.1. Chain analysis of lateness behavior.

likely leads to getting bogged down by irrelevant details, and thus the primary function of the chain analysis is lost. As a clinician becomes more experienced with conducting chains, he or she will develop greater skill to quickly zero in on the important elements. However, it is important to remember that getting quicker with chains is not always the goal.

> Chain analyses can be much shorter in latter sessions when multiple chains have already been completed.

Typical Reasons Why a Problem Isn't Improving

Whenever a problem isn't changing in the intended direction, it is likely a sign that the problem isn't fully understood. At that point, the therapist may go back to the drawing board and look at all parts of the chain in more detail again. In fact, he or she might take even longer with the assessment in order to make sure that the chain of events is fully understood.

If a behavior isn't changing (or has reoccurred after a time), there are several potential reasons.

Previous Chains Were Not Complete or Comprehensive

If this is the case, the target behavior was not fully assessed and important details in the sequence of events are missed. These missed details might be the most critical ones in terms of causes and contributors to the target behavior's reoccurrence. In my experience, details that are more frequently missed include assessment of consequences that may be reinforcing the target behavior, emotions, and secondary targets. For example, a therapist may fail to assess, and thus problem-solve around, the fact that there is an interpersonal reinforcer in the form of caring and soothing from a spouse following a self-injury episode. Thus, despite having conducted many chains previously and worked on several other links, the behavior is unlikely to change unless the contingencies are directed influenced.

Rushing to Solutions

Frequently, therapists notice a dysfunctional link and then stop the chain to offer solutions related solely to that link. This problem is similar to the previous one in that it results in an incomplete assessment. While that solution may work and even sometimes is the best solution for the entire chain of events, rushing to provide a solution usually interferes with a more complete assessment that may highlight other, more critical links upon which to intervene.

Focusing on Noncommon Elements across Chains

Similar to what was discussed in Chapter 5, a therapist can fall into the trap of focusing on a solution that is only relevant to that particular instance of the target behavior. In that case, the solution will not generalize to other situations, and therefore the target behavior is more likely to reoccur. Focusing on unique aspects of the chain will be less successful in the long run and then is likely to also decrease client motivation and hope in treatment.

Solutions Are Too Narrowly Focused

As mentioned in the last chapter, therapists often have their favorite solutions and tend to suggest them even if they don't have a broader impact on the target behavior. Let's say the client in the lateness example above has the thought, "There's no point in getting there on time anyway because treatment isn't helping me with my problems" shortly after getting up. While a focus on modifying that cognition may be warranted (for many reasons), the target behavior of lateness is more strongly controlled by other variables in the chain (e.g., sleep dysregulation). Thus, focusing just on modifying cognition is likely to have little impact on the behavior if the other more critical variables aren't addressed. Behavior is complex and many links in the chain are transactional. That is, each affects the others and the whole is greater than the sum of the parts. Sometimes the therapist has to address multiple links in a chain in order to have effects.

The Core Problem Is Not Addressed

In many circumstances the reason a target behavior is not adequately addressed by a single chain or repeated chains is that a client's "core problem" is not addressed. A "core problem" is a term used to describe a problem that is a common feature across chains of multiple target behaviors (Rizvi & Sayrs, 2018). Linehan (personal communication) recently began using this term in her teaching to help therapists not "lose the forest for the trees" when conducting a chain analysis. That is, sometimes therapists can get mired in the details of the chain to the extent that a central theme goes unassessed. If a core problem is extensively assessed and effective solutions are generated, then it is likely that addressing it will lead to a reduction of target behaviors. If a core problem is not addressed, generated solutions are unlikely to have a lasting impact on behaviors.

In the example of the client's lateness behavior, a therapist might have proposed a solution for a link in the chain that is not related to a core problem. For example, the therapist might have targeted hitting the snooze button so many times and proposed a solution that would make this more difficult (e.g., placing the alarm further away from the bed so that the client has to get up in order to turn it off). Let's assume, however, that this client's sleep difficulties contribute to many problems in her life. She nods off during skills group, she has been late to work as well as excessively sleepy during work, she occasionally takes excess doses of her prescribed stimulant medication to counter her fatigue, and she misses out on important social opportunities because her sleep schedule is out of sync with those of her peers. Thus, the moving-the-alarm-clock solution might address lateness-for-session behavior but not the overarching problem. There might be some short-term benefit to such a change (i.e., it might "work" the following week and lead to the client being on time for the subsequent session). However, it will likely not have a lasting influence if the core problem of sleep dysregulation is not addressed. Thus, the therapist will want to weigh the pros and cons of going for a "quick fix" for the short term versus more immediately addressing the core problem. The latter will have a greater and more sustained impact on the target behavior as well as other problems in the client's life but will take time to establish.

Note that a core problem cannot be identified with a single chain analysis. A problem is only conceptualized as "core" after multiple chains have been conducted that produce similar patterns. Core problems are often harder to see because they can behaviorally manifest in different ways (sleep dysregulation leads to lateness, sleepiness, poor work performance, poor social interactions, etc.). It is often useful to discuss core problems at consultation team meetings so that team members can provide input on their own conceptualizations. Using the case formulation worksheet provided by Rizvi and Sayrs (2018) can also be useful. Of course, not everything involves a core problem and not every chain will be related to one. But if a chain analysis *does* involve a core problem, then the most effective solution will be the one that addresses the common links across multiple chains.

Assessing Behavior That Shows Up Again

In addition to conducting repeated chains on the same behavior that is failing to change, repeated chains may also be done on a behavior that pops up again later in treatment. Usually, a problem behavior that is explicitly targeted in early treatment sessions starts to decrease over time as the client implements the solutions discussed and also increases his or her self-awareness of the behavior. However, in many cases, the target behavior shows up again at a later time and the therapist will want to conduct a chain analysis again. However, at this point, the therapist needs to be eager to understand the context for the behavior reappearing, as it provides information about what may have been missed in previous chains. That is, the question becomes less "How did this behavior occur?" and more "How did this behavior occur *that moment* compared to other moments when it didn't?" With this mind-set, the therapist can home in on the critical variables affecting the presence of the behavior in that instance, while also highlighting all the ways in which the client has improved his or her behavior.

As an example, let's continue with the case of Laurie from Chapter 3. After conducting the original chain analysis in the fifth session, Laurie does not self-injure over the course of the next 8 weeks. During these sessions, the therapist praises this absence, and together they systematically work on increasing more structured activities in the evening to address feelings of loneliness, boredom, and anxiety. This work was based on their shared hypotheses that these emotions were driving the self-injury and that by engaging in behavior that reduces these emotions, the risk of self-injury would be lowered. The therapist also continued to emphasize Laurie's commitment to remain abstinent from self-injury and remembered to do this every week even as the sessions progressed. They also began to make a plan for more directly targeting increasing relationships, both friendships and romantic relationships, since Laurie had identified this as a goal early in treatment and no life-threatening or therapy-interfering behaviors were present.

However, Laurie texted her therapist 2 nights before her 13th therapy session and wrote "I just wanted to give you the heads up that I cut myself tonight. Hope you're not too disappointed." Given that it's later in treatment and that Laurie has been exposed to chain analyses throughout treatment, this presented as an opportunity for Laurie to practice her own self-assessment skills. The therapist also knew that extreme shame could function to shut Laurie down and interfere with successful assessment. Thus, the therapist anticipated that she would have to use a lot of validation and hope generating in combination with her assessment strategies in order to make the chain go smoothly to best identify the next solution. For these reasons, she responded to Laurie the next day by writing back "I can't wait to see you tomorrow so we can figure this all out! If you have time to do a chain analysis before our session, please do one."

Thus, the start of the chain might look quite different later in treatment *and* when a behavior pops up that had been absent for a while. There will likely be disappointment on both the client's and the therapist's parts, and this disappointment has to be acknowledged. For example, the therapist might start the next session by saying:

THERAPIST: I appreciated your heads up a couple of nights ago. It allowed me to experience some of my feelings about it before this session so that now I feel ready to dive in and figure this out. How are you feeling?

LAURIE: I feel terrible. I really wanted to cancel our session today. I just feel like I let you down.

THERAPIST: I appreciate you being so concerned for me, I really do. And I really feel like we're a team here. I want us both to figure out what happened a couple of nights ago since we have made so much progress over that past few months. It's just clear that we have a few remaining kinks to work out.

LAURIE: To say the least.

THERAPIST: Well, hold on, sounds like some self-invalidation or hopelessness there. I get why those might be popping up right now. So we really need to figure out what happened that night so we can assess what needs to be done, OK? Did you get a chance to work on a chain?

Here the therapist is not letting hopelessness derail the need to do the chain. However, she is also using more collaborative "we" language, given that it is later in treatment. In such a chain, she might be looking for the client to generate more herself without as much prompting. Having clients start the chain themselves as homework is one way to encourage this practice.

> Later in treatment, look for the client to generate more of the chain without prompting. Ask clients to start chains as homework.

LAURIE: Yeah, I started to sketch one out. *(Pulls out paper.)*

THERAPIST: Amazing! Really proud of you for starting it! Tell me what you have so far.

LAURIE: OK. I went on a date the night before last that was really horrible. And it was my third horrible date in a row. So after the date, as I was driving home, I was just feeling so hopeless like things would never change, having thoughts like "Why do I even try to improve my life anyway, when nothing will ever work out for me?" So I decided to stop at the drugstore and buy razor blades. Then I went straight home and cut myself in the bathroom, which actually made me feel so much worse. So I regret the whole thing. And I threw out the razor blades, so you don't even have to bother asking me about that!

THERAPIST: Really sorry to hear about the awful date and the cutting. I have to say, though, that you really seem to be getting the essence of chain analysis. Before I ask some more questions about your efforts last night, I'm curious to see if you learned anything from doing the exercise?

LAURIE: Hmm. I think I saw how important those thoughts were. That I was thinking "Why bother?" and kind of discounting all the progress I have made in therapy. I didn't realize I was doing that at the time, but when I wrote this out this morning I saw that more clearly.

THERAPIST: Interesting.

LAURIE: I also saw how it didn't "work" like it used to. I don't think I got any relief from it, the feeling awful just never went away—it just sort of changed focus.

THERAPIST: That highlights a couple of important points. One is that it seems like you have a hypothesis that those hopeless and discounting thoughts were the most important links in driving the self-harm behavior. Is that true?

LAURIE: Yes.

THERAPIST: And the second is that you noticed that you didn't get any relief from the cutting, which is actually great news. It means your cutting wasn't reinforced by a reduction in distress. Now we don't know for sure that this will turn you off from cutting forever, but I think it's really positive because one of the factors that had previously been driving your cutting behavior is not currently there, or at least wasn't there that night.

An astute reader would notice here that the therapist is using sophisticated behavioral language in talking with Laurie about the chain. With clients who have the cognitive capacity to understand such "high-level" communication, this type of language is encouraged. As discussed earlier, a goal with many clients is to get them to learn how to analyze their own behavior in meaningful ways. This means using behaviorally specific language with themselves and not jumping to conclusions about the causes of their behavior.

THERAPIST: So getting back to the chain, let's look again at what you wrote and fill in some details. (Moves seat next to Laurie so that they are both looking at her chain analysis worksheet.) At what point in the sequence of events did the thought of cutting show up? Was it during the drive or anytime before?

LAURIE: It really didn't show up until the drive.

THERAPIST: So not even during the date?

LAURIE: No, I was pretty miserable, but I was more thinking about when will it end, not about cutting.

THERAPIST: OK, so let's take a microscope to that drive. How long was the drive between your date and the drugstore?

LAURIE: Probably just about 5 minutes and then another 2 or 3 minutes to get home.

THERAPIST: This was a pretty short drive and yet a lot happened in your head! You got into your car thinking what about where you were going next?

LAURIE: I don't think I was really thinking about that. I guess I was just in automatic pilot heading home.

THERAPIST: So then describe to me, in more detail, your thoughts during those 5 minutes between the date and the drugstore. Because that's where I think we need to figure out how to do things differently.

This zeroing-in on a piece of the chain and basically ignoring the other parts (note how the therapist has not asked any questions about the date itself) is in contrast to chains that might happen at the beginning of treatment. In those early chains, the therapist doesn't want to make any assumptions about what the most important links are and instead wants to adopt a beginner's mind to get the most accurate picture possible. Later in treatment, when the therapist knows the client and he or her behavior better, the therapist can focus on what he or she believes (with good reason!) to be the essential segment.

From previous chains, including the one from the fifth session, detailed in Chapter 3, the therapist knows that Laurie's emotions and thoughts about her emotions play an important role in eventual cutting, specifically beliefs that self-injury is the only way she can relieve feelings of emotional distress. Now that it's been a while since a self-injurious episode, the therapist wants to understand this connection better.

THERAPIST: One thing I've noticed is that you haven't really mentioned emotions in the chain you wrote up, just that you were feeling hopeless. When you got into the car, what were you feeling?

LAURIE: Definitely hopeless. Also anger, both at the guy for being such an idiot but also at myself.

THERAPIST: Explain that more.

LAURIE: Anger that I'm in this situation at all, I guess. Like if I were a better person, I wouldn't be single right now going on hopeless date after hopeless date.

THERAPIST: Ah, so you were blaming yourself for the situation in part? Do you think shame was there at all? Or anxiety, which you've described as being so devastating in the past? [using knowledge of patterns in the past to drive questions rather than starting with a blank slate]

LAURIE: Definitely blaming myself. And yeah, I guess shame, but I'm not sure I even realized it, if you know what I mean. And I definitely had that agitation that I associate with anxiety like my mind was going a mile a minute and I knew I would have trouble sleeping.

THERAPIST: Ah, so were those thoughts going through your mind too on the drive home—"I'm never going to be able to fall asleep" or something along those lines?

LAURIE: Yes, I think so.

THERAPIST: This has come up before, if you remember. The belief that self-injury is the only thing that can effectively relax you, right?

LAURIE: Yeah (*starting to slump*).

THERAPIST: So it reared its ugly head again. Of course it did—it's been a habit that's developed over years and year, so I'm not surprised. And I think we are so close to successfully addressing it. Just hang in there with me.

LAURIE: You think so? OK, I'm with you.

THERAPIST: So walk me through, as best you can remember, the chain of thoughts in your mind between the date and the drugstore.

LAURIE: "That was horrible. I can't take much more of this. Nothing ever works out for me and I'm going to be alone forever." I started getting really morbid in my head too like "No one would even care if I was alive or dead." I wasn't thinking about killing myself at all; more that, I'll be single forever, I'll never be that person for someone—you know what I mean?

THERAPIST: I think I do. You mean you had the thought that you'll never be someone's most important person?

LAURIE: Yeah, that I'll be the person who dies and isn't found for days.

THERAPIST: I know that thought—it's a side effect of bad dates! And it's really painful to have it. Do you have those sorts of thoughts at other times?

LAURIE: I've definitely had them before, but it's been a while. So this was the first time I remember thinking this in a long time.

THERAPIST: OK, that's helpful to know.

Note how the therapist stays focused on the chain. It would be so easy to get sidetracked here by providing reassurance or by going directly to cognitive modification as a solution and focusing on the evidence for such thoughts. While these might be relevant solutions to suggest later, it is imperative for the therapist to first understand the sequence of events more clearly and also how this sequence relates specifically to the occurrence of self-injury.

THERAPIST: Do you think if you didn't have the "I'm going to die alone" thoughts, you would have gone to the drugstore? [hypothesis testing in order to determine if these thoughts were a critical variable in the chain]

LAURIE: I'm not sure. It was more that I was just sort of thinking that I hate this feeling and that I'm so tired of it all. I just wanted it to go away.

THERAPIST: What is "it"?

LAURIE: Hmm, the hopelessness I guess. And the way it felt in my body. And I saw the drugstore sign coming up and I just decided to buy razors.

THERAPIST: So did you have that thought at all before you saw the drugstore sign on the road?

LAURIE: Not at all.

THERAPISt: And do you think, had you driven down a different road that didn't pass a drugstore, you would have sought out razors?

LAURIE: I can't know for sure, but I'm guessing that the idea wouldn't have crossed my mind really. And I know myself well enough that once I'm home, I'm not going to go out again so I think if I made it home without stopping, I wouldn't have cut.

THERAPIST: I agree. So you saw the drugstore sign, and you said to yourself "I'm going to stop there and get razors." Did any other thoughts enter your mind there? Any thoughts about doing something skillful?

LAURIE: I think I remember thinking that you aren't going to like this but I pushed it out of my mind.

THERAPIST: OK, so you did think of me and your treatment, albeit really briefly. I'd like us to figure out how to elongate the time between thinking about something and doing it so that we have more room to breathe and intervene effectively. [highlights solution to return to] And then you pulled into the drugstore and bought the razors? Anything notable show up?

LAURIE: No, not that I can think of.

THERAPIST: Now, in the past, we discovered that just deciding to self-injure made you feel better and gave you some relief from negative emotions. Did that happen two nights ago? [using knowledge from past chains to make connections]

LAURIE: Yeah, definitely.

THERAPIST: Hmm. So how were you feeling in the drugstore and on the short drive home?

LAURIE: In the drugstore, just sort of determined and focused on getting the razors.

THERAPIST: Interesting. So you weren't thinking hopeless thoughts anymore?

LAURIE: Huh. I can't even remember. If I was, they weren't nearly as intense or stressful.

THERAPIST: And then after you bought the razors and were driving home, what do you think you were thinking and feeling?

LAURIE: The same I think. I was visualizing where I was going to do it. Kind of like seeing the steps in my head before I did it.

THERAPIST: And your emotions then?

LAURIE: Still determined, and probably a bit excited. But like I said, it was totally a let-down, I ended up feeling awful, not better.

THERAPIST: I'm glad about that! And that doesn't change the fact that thinking about self-injury and planning it serves a really important function for you.

LAURIE: Yeah, I suppose.

THERAPIST: So I think I have an idea of the most important links in the chain. Can I list them for you?

LAURIE: Shoot.

THERAPIST: One is, as we just discussed, the link between deciding to self-harm and the immediate relief you feel as a consequence. We need to figure out how to break that link, though I imagine that that's not something for which there is a quick and easy answer. Two, is the link between feeling intensely hopeless and believing that the only thing that will help you is self-harm. I know that isn't true and, if anything, we have learned that it doesn't help you, so we need to find other things to do there. As we've discussed before, you developed tunnel vision and the only thing that occurs to you is self-harm. But we know you are smarter than that and that you have a lot more tools at your disposal. So we need to figure out how to get those alternatives to enter your mind and to increase your willingness to do them. And third is, as I mentioned, increasing the span of time between deciding to do something and doing it— like learning how to be mindful of the urges and just watch them come and go without necessarily acting on them. Do you agree with me?

LAURIE: Yeah, I do. It's not really just about this bad date, is it?

THERAPIST: I agree that the bad date was the prompting event, but it seems like the patterns you have developed are patterns that occur in response to all sorts of negative events in your life, not just bad dates, right?

LAURIE: Right.

This illustration shows what a chain analysis might look like in a later session on a target behavior that has already been assessed. The experienced therapist avoided many of the traps that a more novice therapist might engage in. For example, she does not ask for detail about every link in the chain. Now that she has more knowledge about Laurie and Laurie's history of self-injury, she can more easily zero-in on the parts of the chain that are relevant. However, she still honors the structure and goal of the chain by assessing all of its components. The therapist also avoids rushing to offer solutions before assessing the full sequence. She highlights some potential solutions that are likely helpful (i.e., "We'll need to figure that out."), but makes sure to understand the full story before jumping in. This also provides an example of what it could have looked like for the therapist to focus too narrowly on a less relevant link. That is, Laurie identified driving by the drugstore as a critical variable in this chain and it likely was. When her therapist asked if she would have harmed herself if she didn't pass the drugstore, Laurie responded that it was unlikely. If, in this instance, the therapist had zeroed-in on this variable as an opportunity for solutions, she might have worked with Laurie to find different routes that she could have taken home that would have avoided passing the drugstore. Although it is very likely that this solution would have prevented the self-injury from occurring, it is unlikely that it would have carried over to any many other instances since the circumstances surrounding that drive home were relatively unique (a bad date at that particular location).

In summary, there are several key points for therapists to remember when conducting repeated chains. The first is chains are tools for discovery—not exercises in punishment like the equivalent of writing "I will not self-harm again" 100 times on the blackboard. The therapist needs to approach chain analysis like a detective trying to determine what is missing from the understanding of the problem. This approach highlights for both the therapist and the client the importance of the task. "How is it this behavior is not changing?" is the formative question. Chain analyses remain the primary assessment tool throughout treatment and are used to address that formative question. The therapist and client need to continue to do chain analyses, in some form, for as long as the behavior of interest occurs.

CHAPTER 7

Chains on Thoughts, Urges, and Missing Behaviors

I n teaching the process of chain analyses to students and clinicians, I often focus initially on examples when the target behavior is an overt problem behavior. As the illustrations in this book so far demonstrate, focusing on an observable behavior sets the stage for a comprehensive chain analysis. An overt behavior is usually anchored in time and has a clear start and end, which makes framing the sequence of events around it easier to assess. However, sometimes the problems that need to be targeted are covert behaviors in the form of urges and thoughts. Examples of these covert behaviors include urges to suicide, self-harm, use substances, fantasies about suicide or maladaptive behavior, and rumination. Sometimes the problem is the *absence* of effective behavior, as in the case of someone not practicing skills or other assigned therapy tasks, missing sessions, avoiding doing things that get them closer to their goals, and so on. These urges, thoughts, and missing behaviors frequently are targets of DBT treatment and thus need to be assessed and treated. Oftentimes, chain analyses are still the appropriate method for doing so.

Therapists often don't understand how and when to use chains to assess these behaviors. There is frequently confusion about what type of thought or urge warrants a more thorough assessment. Further, I have noticed that many therapists think a chain is not possible or necessary in these scenarios; instead, the therapists believe either that the situation does not need to be assessed or the situation can be assessed without the structure of the formal chain. One reason for these beliefs is that many therapists don't consider thoughts and urges to be modifiable or necessarily problematic. Therapists frequently have a sense of hopelessness about changing thoughts or urges *or* they are so focused on the fact that an accompanying behavior didn't occur that they lose sight of the fact that thoughts may still be a problem. For example, a client who has stopped self-injuring for months still frequently has fantasies about suicide. The therapist may be so focused on the absence of self-injury that he or she doesn't attend to the fact that fantasizing about suicide is a problem on its own and it increases the risk for suicidal behavior in the future.

DBT is a behavioral treatment and, as such, conceptualizes internal mental activity similarly to observable behaviors. That is, "mental events" occur in a context (antecedents) and have functions (consequences). Thus, understanding the sequence of events leading up to and following a covert behavior can yield just as much information and options for solutions as the assessment of an overt behavior. Similarly, the absence of a needed behavior can be understood in terms of antecedents and consequences as well. In this chapter, I review how and when to use chains to (1) target urges and thoughts and (2) to assess the absence of needed behaviors. The execution of these chains often raises slightly different questions from ones that were covered previously; thus, I use multiple examples to highlight how these assessments can occur.

Targeting Thoughts and Urges

Let me first state the obvious: A therapist does not conduct a chain analysis every time a person has a thought that might be deemed problematic. If that were the case, we would do nothing but chains all the time. So when are thoughts elevated to the point where chain analyses might be considered? This is a difficult question for which there are no "right" answers. The DBT manual does not teach rules about this issue. However, I can suggest some general guidelines that will help clinicians make an informed, and clinically relevant, decision about whether to conduct a chain on a thought, an alternative behavior, or neither. These guidelines are not mutually exclusive categories and, in fact, one thought pattern could be represented by each of them. For example, frequent fantasies about suicide that cause significant subjective distress as well as functional impairment would be an obvious target of a chain analysis even in the absence of a suicide attempt.

Guideline 1: Use the Target Hierarchy

The DBT target hierarchy provides a system of organizing your clinical targets so that you know what to address in any given session. Since individuals in DBT often present with numerous problems, it can be difficult to determine what to prioritize. The hierarchy states that life-threatening behaviors are of utmost priority in DBT and "behaviors" that fall into this category are both overt (e.g., suicide attempts, NSSI) and covert (e.g., suicidal ideation, urges to commit self-harm). Thus, the target hierarchy would suggest that if suicide ideation or urges to suicide occurred in the past week, it would need to be addressed in session, even if other behaviors also occurred (e.g., substance use, binge-eating episodes, avoidance of work). It is not necessarily the case that persistent "low levels" of suicide ideation get targeted in each session. However, if suicide urges are high and/or urges have increased significantly on a certain day, it would be necessary to address them in session.

Similarly, if your top target of treatment is substance use, and a client has thoughts or urges to use substances, even if he or she didn't actually use, the thoughts might be a good candidate for a chain analysis. If a problematic thought is not related to a top target of treatment, then it would likely not rise to the level of importance of a thorough chain analysis.

Guideline 2: Behavior Beats Thoughts about That Behavior

If a person engages in a behavior that is in the highest category of your treatment hierarchy, analysis of that behavior occurs following the steps detailed in previous chapters. Thoughts and urges are then represented as links leading up to, or following, the behavior. In such cases, the thoughts might be a point of intervention or solutions as a way to avoid the target behavior from occurring, but the behavior itself is the anchoring point of the assessment.

Guideline 3: Patterns of Thoughts Are Important for Case Conceptualization and May Represent a "Core Problem"

As discussed in Chapter 6 and in Rizvi and Sayrs (2018), a core problem is one that shows up across multiple chains of different target behaviors. By assessing and addressing a core problem, then, the therapist likely solves problems associated with multiple target behaviors. For example, a client might describe many instances of engaging in "escape fantasies" like imagining quitting her job, being admitted to an inpatient facility, or not leaving her house for days. These escape fantasies function to help her avoid active problem solving, and therefore the antecedents (i.e., problems) are likely to occur again without notable progress. Thus, the therapist might assess a specific instance of recent escape fantasizing using the onset of the fantasy as the target behavior in order to best understand the controlling variables and develop the most appropriate solutions.

Guideline 4: Significant Distress or Negative Consequences Are Associated with the Thought

A chain analysis should be considered if the thoughts themselves are associated with significant distress or impairment. It is likely that a thought that fits this guideline also meets the criteria of the other guidelines listed, but it is also possible that thoughts causing significant subjective distress are not a key target initially. Alternatively, a client might have his or her behavior under control but the experience of certain thoughts represents a problem. For example, a client who has distressing thoughts related to her appearance ("I'm ugly") may not notice a significant impact on her overt behavior but she experiences these thoughts as out of control and harmful. Conducting a chain analysis on an instance where the thought popped up would likely yield valuable information about what contexts or situations are antecedents to the "I'm ugly" thought as well as what an immediate consequence of that thought might be (e.g., client shuts down and doesn't engage in conversation with partner).

Orienting Rationales

With these guidelines in mind, a therapist who decides to target a thought or urge will follow much of the same procedures as with chains of overt behaviors. As with chains of overt behaviors, the clinician often has to orient the client to the procedures and "sell" them as relevant and necessary. Thus, the reasons for conducting standard chains on thoughts and urges need to be clear to therapists and clients alike. First, as mentioned, thoughts such as suicide ideation and urges to self-harm fall under the target category of "life-threatening behaviors" in DBT, and thus need to be targeted and reduced before moving on to other problems on the client's treatment hierarchy. Second, even if the thoughts and urges are not life-threatening, their very presence often increases the risk that the person will engage in the associated behavior in the future (even if it was not present that time). For example, someone with a substance abuse history who has been sober for several months reports an uptick in thoughts about drinking in recent days. Even if he has not consumed any alcohol, these thoughts would definitely serve as a red flag and a major risk factor for drinking in the future. Thus, assessing the circumstances leading to the occurrence of the thoughts, as well as the consequences of the thoughts, are incredibly relevant for treatment. A third reason is that conducting chains on thoughts and urges allows for opportunities to figure out and strengthen what helped the person to *not* engage in a particular behavior. That is, instead of only focusing on the thoughts as a problem to be solved, a therapist can also focus on the fact that the accompanying behavior did not occur and attempt to assess the protective factors, or skills used, that can be reinforced and strengthened. These reasons can all be used to "sell" the client on the importance of the chain in this scenario.

Once it has been determined that a thought or urge would benefit from a chain analysis, in many ways they proceed like every other chain that has been discussed thus far. The thought can be identified as the target behavior and described behaviorally and topographically (e.g., "I had thoughts and images about consuming a bottle of pills that lasted for about 30 minutes while I was lying alone in bed"). A prompting event is identified (e.g., "A couple hours prior, I had a negative interaction with my best friend and she said that she needed a break from me for a while"). Links between the prompting event and the problem behavior are described in terms of emotions, other thoughts, and behaviors. Factors that made the client more vulnerable to the prompting event on that particular day are elicited, if relevant. Finally, consequences of the thoughts themselves are assessed. Additionally, other strategies to keep the client engaged and motivated, such as appropriate orientation, dialectics, validation, reciprocal communication, and irreverence, are emphasized as before.

Challenges with This Type of Chain Analysis

Although the structure of chain analyses with mental events remains the same, there are frequently a couple of distinct challenges in conducting them. The first potential challenge is specifically identifying the target behavior and anchoring it in time. The second potential challenge involves the assessment of consequences. I next describe these two challenges in more detail and highlight ways to address them.

Identifying the Specific Target Behavior

Usually people don't experience a discrete thought unrelated to other thoughts flooding their mind that they can easily identify and anchor in time. Therefore, it can often be difficult to identify *the* thought that is the target or even when that thought first occurred. It might be easier when the thought is particularly notable, as in the case of suicide urges when a therapist can ask, "When did the thought of killing yourself first enter your mind," but more difficult with thoughts that don't stand out in the moment. For example, most people would struggle with identifying the very first thought that set off an hour of rumination. The important strategy here is not to get lost in the weeds. A therapist may need to start with approximations in order to get relevant information to help effect change later. Questions like "When did you first notice that thought?" or "What were you doing when that urge showed up?" will aid in getting a sense of the timeline.

Consequences of Thoughts and Urges

The fact that thoughts can have consequences that control their occurrence is sometimes difficult to grasp. Since the behavior is internal, it can be difficult for clients (and therapists) to see direct connections between the thoughts and internal and external consequences. However, when assessed, clients will frequently state that thoughts about engaging in problematic behavior often make them feel better and/or reduce distress. Importantly, the thoughts or fantasies about engaging in problematic behavior often have a particular *function* as avoidance of more active and effective problem solving. Thus, the consequences of the thoughts are frequently important controlling variables and can also highlight some of the reasons why changing thoughts, like other behaviors, can be so difficult.

The clinician conducting a chain on thoughts has to carefully assess the immediate consequences of them. It is necessary to focus on internal consequences (e.g., "What emotions did you have immediately after that thought?"; "What else did you think immediately after that first urge?";

"What did you feel in your body when you noticed that thought?"), as well as on external consequences (e.g., "What did you do immediately after that thought went through your mind?"). Understanding the consequences of thoughts and urges might not occur with one chain but may develop after noting particular patterns. The therapist needs to wonder what the thoughts are doing for the person, that is, what function do they have that make it more likely that the thoughts will reoccur.

Example of a Chain Analysis of Suicidal Ideation

I next show what a chain analysis of a covert behavior could look like. The client, Angelica, is a 20-year-old college student. The following chain analysis occurred 6 weeks into treatment. At the prior week's skills group, Angelica had disclosed to the group leaders that she was "feeling suicidal" at the end of group. The skills leaders assessed for risk and made a plan with Angelica that involved practicing several skills, getting in touch with her best friend, and reaching out to her therapist. At the subsequent session, the therapist noted on the diary card that the day of skills group (Tuesday), Angelica's ratings of suicide ideation (SI) were 5 out of 5 but there was no self-harm reported. On the other days of the week, suicide ideation was rated as 0, 1, or 2. Thus, Tuesday's suicide ideation was the top target for the session.

THERAPIST: OK, so last week during skills group you were really distressed, you were having some suicidal ideation, and you spoke with the co-leader after group to assess your risk and make a safety plan. In our session today I'd like to discuss exactly what those feelings and thoughts were, what led up to them, and how to prevent things from reaching that point in the future. [targeting and orienting to chain]

ANGELICA: OK. But you know I didn't do anything.

THERAPIST: I do know and I'm so, so proud of you for having high intensity thoughts and urges without engaging in suicidal behavior. That's part of what I want to figure out—how you managed these thoughts in more effective ways. That said, I still think it's a problem that you so frequently have thoughts about killing yourself, even if you don't actually do anything, don't you?

ANGELICA: Yeah, I guess so.

THERAPIST: I would prefer for you to have tough days without also having thoughts about wanting to be dead! So what happened on Tuesday?

ANGELICA: I'd made a phone call right before group to this guy I liked and he rejected me.

THERAPIST: And after that call is when you started thinking about killing yourself? Was that the first time the SI came up on Tuesday? Immediately after the call?

ANGELICA: Yeah. And then it sort of grew over time.

THERAPIST: So tell me more about the SI. What form did it take? [assessing target behavior]

ANGELICA: What do you mean?

THERAPIST: How do you know you had SI at a 5? Was it thoughts, feelings, or what? Can you describe that to me? [assessing target behavior]

ANGELICA: Yeah, I guess it was intense thoughts. Like "I hate my life and I just want it to be over." I was just feeling a lot of things and thought everything would be better if I were dead.

THERAPIST: How long did that thought last? Did it just flit into your brain and out again or did it stick around?

ANGELICA: Definitely stuck around. It probably lasted for most of the evening.

THERAPIST: And did it get to the point where you were thinking specifics about what you might do to kill yourself?

ANGELICA: Well, I knew I had to go to group, so it was more like I was thinking that after group I could go to sleep and maybe not wake up.

THERAPIST: Did you plan anything with regard to that? Like getting pills or something?

ANGELICA: No, that was as far as I got.

THERAPIST: OK. Well I'm really glad it didn't get farther than that. So let's look at the whole chain of events, thoughts, and feelings that led up to the SI and what followed after. So the call was at what time? [identifying prompting event]

ANGELICA: I called him at 5:45 while I was walking to group, and I sat outside and talked to him for about 5 minutes.

THERAPIST: OK, let's see what was going on before, and then we'll look at what happened after. What were you doing right before the call?

ANGELICA: Well, I was planning on calling him because I'd been thinking about calling him all day. I actually called my friend and asked for her advice. She told me it was important for me to be honest with him.

THERAPIST: When was that?

ANGELICA: Around 4:30.

THERAPIST: What feelings were you having before calling him?

ANGELICA: Anxious, obviously. I was thinking "What will he say? Is he gonna reject me?" And there was also fear of change.

THERAPIST: Fear that if you call him, the situation between the two of you wouldn't stay the same?

ANGELICA: Yeah.

THERAPIST: You had about an hour between calling your friend and calling him. What was going on then? Any thoughts about suicide?

ANGELICA: No. I was busy with homework at home and talking to my mom.

THERAPIST: OK, and how was that going?

ANGELICA: I was anxious, thinking about making the call, but I was getting it done. I was getting it done but I don't think I was really focused on it.

THERAPIST: And on your diary card it showed that that this was the day after you had only slept 3 hours, right?

ANGELICA: Yeah.

THERAPIST: OK, so there may have been some other factors that might've impacted how you reacted in this situation, made you more vulnerable, and why you ended up thinking about suicide [remaining focused on suicidal thinking as the problem behavior]. Irregular sleep is one. Were there any other factors at play here? [identifying vulnerability factors]

ANGELICA: I wasn't feeling well, my cold had reached a peak.

THERAPIST: OK. Anything else? Did you have anything stressing you out that day?

ANGELICA: No, not really. But really, his rejecting me felt really big. I think I would have felt the way I did even if I had slept better.

THERAPIST: I can see that. I'm sure being sick and tired didn't help the situation, but this event was pretty big and the rejection struck you really hard, and so that event seems more critical than the vulnerabilities here. So you had all of these thoughts and anxieties. When did you decide to call him and tell him about your feelings?

ANGELICA: About 5:30. I couldn't take the anxiety anymore, so I was thinking I needed to find out "now" otherwise I wouldn't be able to focus on anything during group.

THERAPIST: So you were feeling an urgent need to resolve this before group, or you wouldn't be able to pay attention?

ANGELICA: Kind of, yeah. I was originally planning to call after group, but then I was like "I can't wait."

THERAPIST: OK, so then you call him. What happened next?

ANGELICA: Rejection.

THERAPIST: Before that. How did you start the conversation?

ANGELICA: I told him, "I know we agreed to keep it casual, but I've realized that I really love you and if we could be a 'serious thing' I would really like it," and he said, "I'm sorry, but I don't feel the same way."

THERAPIST: Oof, that is rough! How did you feel then?

ANGELICA: Awful. Just so ashamed.

THERAPIST: I get that. These experiences are so painful—you put yourself out there in a really bold and important way and I'm proud of you for that even though it didn't turn out how you hoped. How did the call end?

ANGELICA: I just sort of shut down and said something stupid probably like "OK, well see you around" and then hung up.

THERAPIST: It's hard to process that all in such a short time. How long did the phone call last do you think?

ANGELICA: Honestly, probably only a couple of minutes. I plunged right into the discussion because I was feeling anxious and then when he said that, I just got off the phone as quickly as possible. And then I immediately started judging myself, thinking, "Why did I call?"; "Why was I feeling those things?"; "I should've known better than to call"; "I should've just kept things the same."

THERAPIST: OK, so let's say the prompting event for the suicidal thoughts was the rejection. Immediately after that you had these thoughts.

Let's also add the feelings you had after the call. You mentioned rejection. What else were you feeling at that moment? [assessing links]

ANGELICA: Feeling inadequate, like there's something wrong with me.

THERAPIST: Those are still thoughts. Can you think of feelings or emotions that go along with those kinds of thoughts?

ANGELICA: Probably shame and embarrassment.

THERAPIST: Yeah, that's what I would feel too. And those are really painful emotions. And when did the SI show up?

ANGELICA: Right around then. I'm walking to group having these thoughts and feelings and then the "I just want to be dead" thoughts showed up.

THERAPIST: Now this might be a strange question, but I want to zero in here for a minute. You're walking to group, you just got off the phone with this guy, you are feeling intense shame and embarrassment, and then having thoughts about wanting to be dead. What consequences did those thoughts have?

ANGELICA: Huh?

THERAPIST: I know it sounds strange. But if we think about the thoughts of wanting to be dead as the problem behavior here, there were likely immediate consequences, even though you might not have been aware of them at the time. What do you think happened to your thoughts or feelings when you started thinking "I wish I was dead"?

ANGELICA: Hmm, I'm not sure.

THERAPIST: Let me throw something out there and see if you agree. Sometimes when we have thoughts, even if the thoughts themselves are distressing, they function to help us avoid thinking about something that feels even worse. In this case, I'm wondering if you started thinking more about being dead than you were thinking about the rejection.

ANGELICA: Ah, I see what you mean. You're probably right. I started thinking about getting through group and going home to my bed and hoping I wouldn't wake up.

THERAPISt: Right! So your brain was actually trying to solve the problem in a way. The problem of being really agitated, ashamed, and embarrassed. The problem is that it gave you a very short-term ineffective solution rather than helping you cope with the distress is a more effective way. See what I mean?

ANGELICA: Yeah, I get it.

THERAPIST: This also means that the thoughts are "doing something for you," which is why they are difficult to change. But we can do it, I'm pretty confident about this. In looking over this whole chain there is a lot going on, and this gave me a better picture. Hopefully, it gave you a clearer picture too.

Commentary

In this chain (illustrated in Figure 7.1), Angelica's highest order target was the life-threatening behavior of SI in the past week, and thus needed to be assessed and treated. Here I demonstrated how the therapist used a standard, relatively straightforward chain analysis to assess the SI. As previously discussed, the therapist had to work a bit harder to identify the specific problem behavior and the consequences, or functions, of the SI and used some of the strategies described in order to do so. The therapist remained steadfast in pursuing the thoughts about suicide as the target behavior and highlighted the importance of doing so.

Targeting the Absence of Effective Behaviors with Chain Analysis

In addition to conducting chains on thoughts or urges, another topic of chain analysis that might need to be carefully assessed is the absence of effective behaviors. Many therapy-interfering behaviors could be classified in this way. For example, missing sessions, not doing homework, or failing to do other therapy tasks are frequently instances of the client not engaging in effective behavior. Other target behaviors might fall into this category as well, such as a client with an eating disorder not eating at a specified time or a client with social anxiety not attending classes. Thus, the absence of effective behavior is a frequent disussion in treatment across all sorts of target problems and would often benefit from a more careful assessment of causes and consequence. However, a common question with this type of chain is "What exactly is the target behavior?"

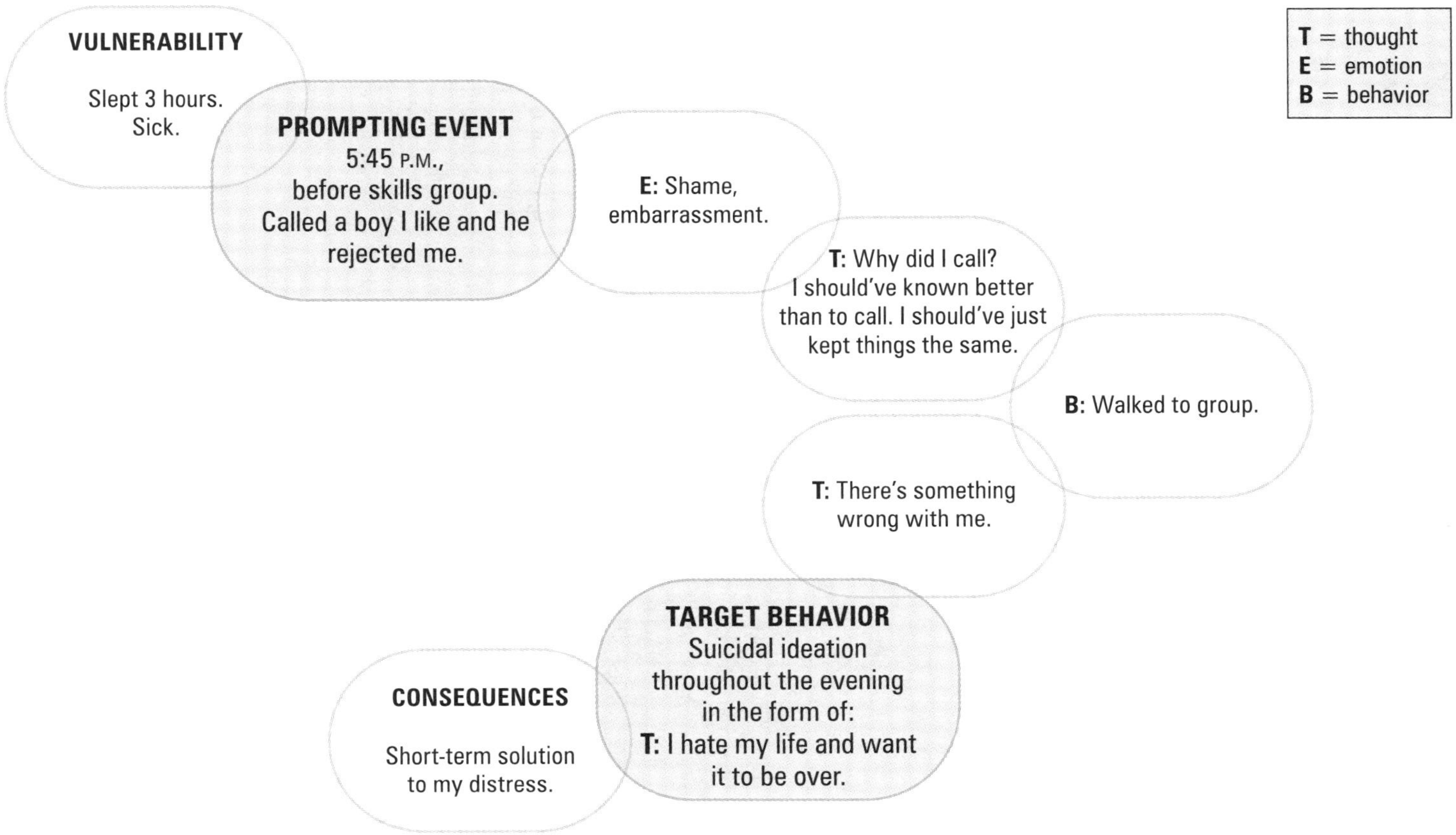

FIGURE 7.1. Chain analysis of suicide ideation.

Legend:
- **T** = thought
- **E** = emotion
- **B** = behavior

VULNERABILITY
Slept 3 hours.
Sick.

PROMPTING EVENT
5:45 P.M.,
before skills group.
Called a boy I like and he
rejected me.

E: Shame,
embarrassment.

T: Why did I call?
I should've known better
than to call. I should've just
kept things the same.

B: Walked to group.

T: There's something
wrong with me.

TARGET BEHAVIOR
Suicidal ideation
throughout the evening
in the form of:
T: I hate my life and want
it to be over.

CONSEQUENCES
Short-term solution
to my distress.

149

Missing Links Analysis

This is such a common problem in treatment that when Linehan was revising her skills manual, in addition to including the skill of chain analysis, she also developed the "missing links" assessment. Briefly, missing links analysis involves running through a series of questions in sequence when effective behavior is missing in order to identify a specific problem to be addressed and solved. From Linehan (2015), these questions are:

1. "Did I know what effective behavior was needed or expected?"
2. "Was I willing to do what was needed?"
3. "Did the thought of doing what was needed or expected enter my mind?"
4. "What got in the way of doing what was needed or expected right away?"

If a question is answered "Yes," the analysis proceeds to the next question. An answer "No" at any point indicates the potential controlling variable for the problem and then leads to problem solving. This analysis can potentially solve the problem on its own. For example, if the client indicates that he didn't know what effective behavior was needed when he was asked to complete a diary card, then the therapist might instruct him about how to complete the diary card more fully and make sure that the client clearly understands the procedure. If that was the primary problem, now that he understands how to fill in the diary card, he will do it. If the problem arose in the third question (the client didn't think about it), the therapist might work to determine how best to cue the client to remember. Sometimes, a simple reminder system or phone alert can then elicit the needed behavior in a reliable way. However, it is also likely that the missing links analysis yields information about a more complicated pattern of behavior that then might be an appropriate target for the chain analysis.

To help navigate these murky decisions, I created a therapist flowchart (see Figure 7.2). This flowchart can help the therapist identify whether there is something that would be helpful to target via a chain analysis when a client does not engage in an effective or important behavior. In such a case, the first step is usually just to ask, "What happened?" or "What got in the way?" in order to get a brief description of the circumstances. The therapist needs to be careful to not let this question lead to

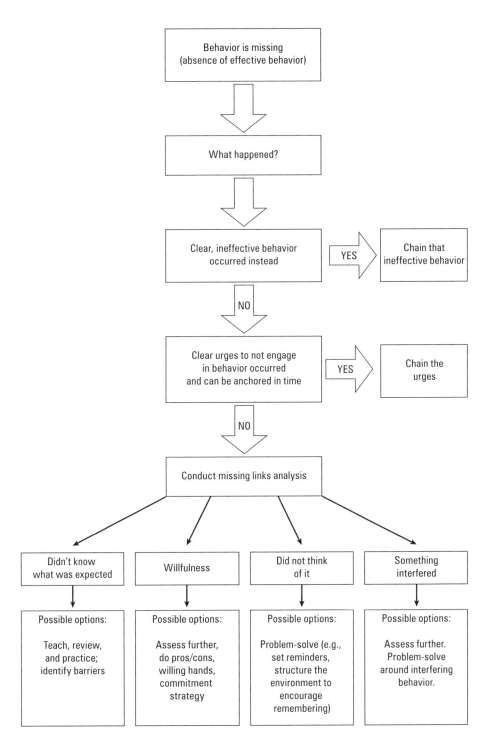

FIGURE 7.2. Analysis flowchart.

a lengthy story or a discussion about other things. Instead, the focus is clearly on a particular instance. So the therapist might say, "You didn't show up for group last week. What happened?" in order to get a response like "I was feeling overwhelmed by my day and just thought I deserved a night 'off,' so I went home instead of driving to group." Once some information is gathered about the circumstances surrounding the absence of the effective behavior, the rest of the flowchart can fall into place.

For instance, the response to the initial question of "What happened?" might lead to the identification of a clear *ineffective* behavior that occurred instead of the desired behavior. If that happens, usually the easiest, and most clinically relevant, thing to do would be to proceed with a chain analysis of that ineffective behavior. For example, imagine that a client missed a therapy session because she impulsively agreed to go on a date at the same time as her scheduled session. In this case, agreeing to go on the date (and then going) might be framed as the target behavior in a chain analysis. Similarly, texting to cancel one's appointment and then turning the phone off so as not to see any response might be the appropriate target behavior when the problem was missing the session.

Of course, there are also many instances in which there is no clear ineffective behavior that interfered. Rather, the interference is more ambiguous or difficult to isolate. The response above of "I was feeling overwhelmed by my day and just thought I deserved a night 'off,' so I went home instead of driving to group" is such an example. In that response, it is hard to identify one clear problem that can be targeted. Using the flowchart as our guide, we might respond "No" to "Clear Ineffective Behavior Occurred Instead" and so we move on to the next step. Here, we want to see whether we can determine if there were urges to not engage in effective behavior and if those urges can be anchored in time. These urges could be assessed with a question like "When did the thought of *not* doing [effective behavior] first enter your mind?" If the client can identify a particular start point of that thought, it is possible for a chain to be conducted with that thought as the target behavior. For example, the client could respond, "I was at work, feeling miserable and tired, and right as I was getting ready to leave for the day, I had the thought 'I want to go home instead of going to group.' Once that thought came in my mind, I just went with it." The therapist can then assess the sequence of events leading up to that thought as well as the consequences. Subsequently, the therapist and client can work together to identify more adaptive solutions for similar events in the future.

If a clear ineffective target behavior was not present and urges to avoid the effective behavior cannot be identified or isolated in time, the time might be right for a missing links analysis. This analysis will then help the therapist zero-in on what the primary issue is that controlled the behavior. For example, let's say the missing behavior being targeted is the client not doing the assigned diary card during the week. The missing links analysis can help the therapist figure out what the primary controlling variable for the missing diary card was and then potentially lead to a chain analysis or perhaps lead to a "quick" solution. For example, if the client knew what was needed but then didn't think about the diary card once during the week, the therapist can help to solve the problem by working with the client to determine ways to remember the diary card (e.g., reminders, setting up alerts on one's phone or computer, placing the card in a particular location). If the missing links analysis identifies will-fulness/avoidance as getting in the way of the behavior ("I remembered it, but then didn't want to do it"), the therapist can assess this avoidance more thoroughly in order to determine what can be changed for the future. Sometimes going through the missing links analysis leads to the identification of an ineffective behavior that was previously not identified. For example, a client does not do his assigned homework of calling to make a psychiatry appointment and says that he just "totally spaced it." Going through the missing links, the therapist uses the questions and finds out that, in fact, the client did think about calling the psychiatrist, but then had the thought that he didn't really need medications after all. The therapist will then want to assess this thought, and associated thoughts, that interfere with him being effective in the situation.

I also want to emphasize here that not every example of a missing effective behavior would necessarily lead to a standard chain analysis. An experienced therapist may be able to drop the structure of the chain and instead assess the sequence of events that occurred around the avoidance behavior without a clear definition of the target behavior. This strategy can be especially helpful when the avoidance behavior is of long duration and somewhat diffuse. For example, a client with a long-standing pattern of extreme food restriction behavior was assigned the task of eating three meals a day at appointed times. The following week, the client reported not eating the lunch meal at all. The therapist might ask, "OK, yesterday, at noon, what happened that you didn't eat?," to which the client responds, "I didn't want to." Rather than try to zero-in on a particular urge or alternate behavior that could take some time and likely not yield too much helpful information, the therapist could instead say, "OK, walk me through this a bit. Tell me more about what happened yesterday that led to you not eating at noon." The focus is still on a clear, behavioral assessment of the factors that contribute to the absence of effective behavior.

Example of How to Structure a Chain Analysis of Missing Previous Session

For this example, I am not going to detail all the steps of the chain because that has already been thoroughly reviewed. Instead, I'm going to demonstrate how to anchor a chain analysis and orient the client to one when the targeted behavior is the absence of effective behavior. In this case, the therapist is targeting a missed session from the week prior. The client, Marcus, was a 45-year-old, unmarried, unemployed man who was in his fifth week of treatment. At the first session, he readily committed to all of DBT's agreements including participating in the treatment for a full year by attending both individual and group and giving up self-injury (which he had a relatively minimal history of, having only done it four times in his life). Marcus experienced severe depression and spent most of his day isolated at home in his apartment watching TV. He was scheduled to meet with his therapist at 5:00 P.M. on Tuesday, but called her a half-hour prior to the session to say that he couldn't come because he was sick. The therapist attempted to assess further and get him to come in, but he repeatedly said he was "not well" and that he would see her the following week. Something about his tone of voice and evasiveness made the therapist question if he was really physically ill. Thus, the therapist wanted to assess the therapy-interfering behavior of missing therapy at the subsequent session. After a check-in and review of the diary card, the following occurred:

THERAPIST: I wanted to check in with you about last week and our missed session.

MARCUS: Yeah, I was sick. Sorry I couldn't make it.

THERAPIST: I was sorry too. I was looking forward to seeing you. Can you tell me a bit more about what happened? [first step of flowchart]

MARCUS: What do you mean? I was sick!

THERAPIST: Oh, I know. Let me back up. We still don't know each other very well and we've only seen each other for four sessions. You canceling last week might just be a totally one-off thing and it won't come up again. But I'm also wondering if there might have been some avoidance going on—like maybe you didn't really feel like coming in for therapy, so you called to cancel without explaining what was really happening. And maybe this sort of thing also happens in other areas of your life. So I'm wondering if we could just spend a few minutes talking about last week so that I have a better sense of what was going on and we can figure out whether we need to do anything differently going forward. Or not. Know what I mean? [orienting and providing rationale]

MARCUS: *(looking down, embarrassed)* Yeah, I guess so.

THERAPIST: So can you tell me more about last Tuesday? When did you decide to cancel? [anchoring in time and asking specific, rather than open-ended, question]

MARCUS: Probably right before I called you.

THERAPIST: So about 4:30?

MARCUS: Yeah, I had been going back and forth in my head about whether I should come in for hours and finally I just decided and called you.

THERAPIST: Oh, OK. So when did you first start thinking about canceling?

MARCUS: Probably when I woke up that morning.

THERAPIST: Wow, OK! What time was that?

MARCUS: Probably around 11:30 or so.

THERAPIST: And what were you feeling then?

MARCUS: Blah.

THERAPIST: Hmm, "blah" can mean a lot of things. What did it mean for you that day?

MARCUS: Depressed, sort of achy. Not wanting to do anything.

THERAPIST: OK, I'm hearing a lot of depression sorts of things. I'm wondering, do you think you were physically ill that day?

MARCUS: Mmm, maybe not.

THERAPIST: So there may have also been some lying behavior happening that day? In terms of what you said to me over the phone? [nonjudgmental stance—just describing]

MARCUS: I guess so, but I really wasn't feeling well.

THERAPIST: True, I get that you were feeling really down and depressed. And that sort of not feeling well is the perfect time to come to a therapy session, right? The more you avoid therapy when you're feeling that way, the less helpful I'm going to be.

MARCUS: Yeah, OK.

THERAPIST: So walk me through the sequence of events *(The therapist stands up and goes to the whiteboard to start drafting this up.)* You wake up at 11:30 and almost immediately feel depressed and have thoughts that you don't want to do anything, right? *(Marcus nods.) (The therapist puts this at the start of the chain.)* And at 4:30 P.M., you call me to cancel. *(The therapist puts this toward the end of the chain as the target behavior.)* Now we'll go through and fill in all the blanks, OK?

Commentary

By following the flowchart, the therapist is anchoring the assessment to the behavior of calling to cancel since that was rooted in time and was directly related to the behavioral absence of not attending the session. Using other strategies discussed previously, the therapist orients Marcus to the purpose of the chain and also connects the missing-session behavior to other problems in the client's life, thus hopefully improving the client's willingness to see this as a problem that needs to be assessed and solved in a collaborative manner.

There might be other scenarios in which a client has a very similar chain but doesn't call to cancel, instead he just "no shows" the session. Following the flowchart, in that scenario, the chain could be anchored to the point at which he made the clear decision not to attend (target behavior) and the therapist can similarly start from the point at which he first thought of not attending (prompting event—or something external that preceded this first thought). Or if there was no clear decision, the therapist could then assess for when the urges to not attend first appeared and see if they could be targeted with a chain.

How to Structure a Chain Analysis of Avoidance Behavior

Now imagine a similar scenario with Marcus in which the issue wasn't that he missed a session. Instead, he stayed in his bed all day feeling depressed but did not miss any appointments or experience dire negative consequences because he had nothing scheduled that day. However, his staying in bed all day was a target for treatment because it was a representative behavior of his severe depression which was a top quality-of-life-interfering problem. The therapist had been focusing on behavioral activation strategies including increasing structure and mastery experiences and decreasing avoidance and staying-in-bed behaviors. In this case, the problem behavior is a bit more difficult to define and anchor in time. Marcus says he woke up and then stayed in bed all day, getting up only to eat sometimes and use the bathroom. What might be the most appropriate way to assess this event and could a chain analysis be a helpful tool?

Using the flowchart, after getting a brief description of what happened, the therapist would determine if there was a clear ineffective behavior that occurred and could be anchored in time. In this particular case, the ineffective behavior might be conceptualized as "staying-in-bed behavior." Marcus says he stayed in bed all day which, on first appearance, might seem difficult to anchor in time. However, it is possible to find ways to anchor it more specifically. Theoretically, one could target the first minute after waking up in which he likely makes some decisions to stay in bed rather than to get out of bed. The difficulty with focusing on this minute is that there is likely only so much information that can be assessed within that 1 minute of time. Another possibility would be to assess the first time he got out of bed to go to the bathroom or eat and then focus on the moment he went *back* to bed that first time as the target behavior. In such a scenario, the focus is on the decision to get back into bed rather than stay out of bed, and by assessing that sequence, the therapist is striving to figure out ways to alter the chain of events in the future at an early point. In both of these cases, the therapist is using staying-in-bed behavior as the clear ineffective behavior to be targeted and assessed.

In this chapter, I reviewed examples and guidelines for how to do a chain analysis when the target behavior is less clearly defined. Working with thoughts and urges as target behaviors is necessary in many cases, but first a therapist has to learn how to navigate the unique factors associated with his or her assessment. What to do when a behavior that is needed did not occur poses its own assessment challenges. Clinicians can use the guidelines presented in this chapter to work with all these behaviors in the same way as overt problem behaviors.

CHAPTER 8

Chain Analyses in Consultation Teams, Skills Training, and Phone Coaching

The major portion of this book has intentionally focused on the use of chain analyses in the context of an individual therapy session. Given the time needed to conduct adequate chain analyses and their role in case conceptualization and treatment planning, it makes sense for chains to be largely in the domain of individual therapy with the primary therapist. However, if chain analyses are viewed as the primary assessment tool in DBT more broadly, then we also have to consider the three other modes of DBT therapy as situations in which the need for chain analyses might arise. In this chapter, I describe the sorts of situations that might call for a chain analysis in consultation teams, skills training, and phone coaching, as well as modifications that would need to be made in order to efficiently and effectively conduct them across these different contexts. In doing so, I introduce the idea of a "macro chain" and how it might be used in multiple contexts.

Micro Chains and Macro Chains

In DBT, the framework of the chain analysis provides a guide for how we assess everything. That is, the fundamental assumption in DBT, and behaviorism more generally, is that every behavior exists in the context of a sequence of events. These events are made up of thoughts, emotions, and behaviors of self and others. Some of these events, or *links*, play an important role in the presence of the target behavior and some do not. The former are often referred to as *controlling variables,* which we strive to identify and change in order to influence the presence of the target behaviors. The previous seven chapters have illustrated ways in which we conduct more formal chains in individual therapy in order to identify the controlling behaviors and implement solutions that will have the most impact on changing the target behavior. Oftentimes, these assessments occur at the *micro* level, meaning that we attempt to determine every link so that the entire sequence is well known to both the client and the therapist. These thorough chains are frequently needed in individual therapy to really understand a problem behavior that has been occurring for a long time or is impervious to change attempts. However, there are also less formal assessment strategies that incorporate the chain framework, and these informal strategies can be flexibly applied across situations and settings. Sometimes a *macro* approach is warranted, that is, zooming out to get a sense of the major components of the chain without attending to every single link. These "macro chains" may be done when there isn't time to do an in-depth chain, a fine-point analysis is not needed, or when broad strokes might provide valuable information. In essence, you don't need to conduct a full-length, link-by-link, moment-by-moment chain in every circumstance.

Learning to differentiate between when a micro chain versus a macro chain is called for is a skill that develops over time as it is largely context-dependent. Commonalities between the two include the five components (vulnerability, prompting event, links, target behavior, consequences), a linear sequential focus, and an attempt to identify the controlling variables that are most receptive to intervention. In terms of differences, a macro chain is going to take far less time to complete. The therapist may not attempt to understand every single step in the chain and might instead let some unanswered questions go by in the service of gaining an understanding of the broad strokes.

To illustrate, Figure 8.1 shows a sample chain analysis for an instance of group lateness behavior by a client. The left-hand side demonstrates what a standard chain might look like, while the right-hand side demonstrates a macro-level chain.

Macro chains are more frequently used in the three other modes of DBT treatment because there are often higher-order targets in these contexts. The consultation team is the mode in which chains might be most often used, after individual therapy. The focus in that context is

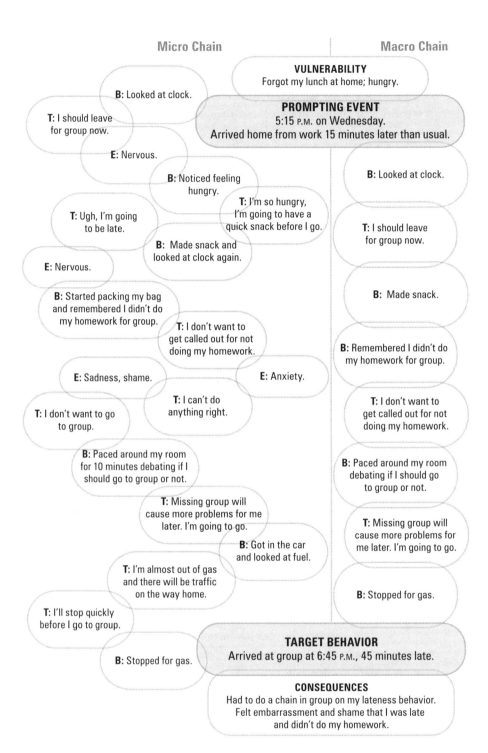

FIGURE 8.1. Micro- versus macro-chain analysis on group lateness.

on building therapist adherence to the treatment and reducing burnout. Sometimes chain analyses can help with both of these targets, but just as often other strategies are used. In skills training, the primary focus is on increasing skills acquisition. A chain might be used in the context of skills training when it helps in that mission and/or when it is designed to reduce a therapy-interfering behavior that gets in the way of skills acquisition. On phone calls, the targets are to reduce suicide crises, increase skills generalization, and decrease therapy relationship conflict. In addition, phone calls are meant to be brief. Thus, chains are used sparingly during phone calls. I describe examples of chains in each of these modes below.

Use of Chain Analysis in Consultation Teams

The team consultation meeting is an important context for chain analyses and they are frequently employed there. Consultation teams can provide opportunities for role plays in order for therapists to hone their skills in a situation in which taking risks is encouraged and straightforward feedback is provided. This is true for the practice of chain analyses as well.

For example, long ago, it became an informal rule in team consultation meetings that therapists would conduct chain analyses on any late members. The idea is that this would give therapists opportunities to practice doing chain analyses in a short period of time with a real-life situation as well as provide a consequence for the latecomer. Unfortunately, what I have observed is that this has become a rote exercise for many teams; very few people see them as an opportunity to practice, learn, and improve. Below, I talk about how to improve the practice of conducting macro chains on lateness behavior in teams and also how to use chains in teams more broadly and not just on lateness.

Orienting to Chain Analysis in Teams

As with chains in individual therapy, orientation to the rationale of conducting chains in teams is extremely important. The more individual members find chains helpful, informative, and related to improvements in therapy with clients, the more likely they are to see them as something they are excited to continue to practice in team. In a sense, there are two separate rationales for chains in team, both of which can be emphasized: one is to improve the understanding of a therapist's own behavior and the other is to improve the skill of conducting chain analyses. The recipient of a chain can benefit as well as the person who practices conducting the chain. Initially, the rationale might need to be provided by the team leader, but over time other team members can rise to the occasion of "selling" chains to fellow members if necessary.

Besides lateness, other behaviors that might prompt chains in team include team-interfering behaviors such as a therapist not doing something that he or she committed to doing for the team, taking phone calls during a team meeting, or missing the team meeting entirely. A therapist might bring up his or her own behavior as a problem for which he or she needs help with the team and by doing so, "volunteer" it for chain analyses. For example, a therapist may highlight something problematic that happened in a session (e.g., laughing along with the client when the client jokes about her own suicide attempt; not asking for a commitment to reduce drinking behavior). The therapist wants help from the team in figuring out how it happened and how to prevent it from happening again. At other times, the team may bring up a behavior of a therapist that is in need of assessment and problem solving. For example, an astute team member may notice that the team has discussed the need for one of the therapists to do in-session exposures with a client for several weeks, but the therapist has yet to institute the procedure. The missing links analysis, discussed in Chapter 7, may be used to identify what is getting in the way of the therapist implementing exposure, which may yield a specific target behavior to chain.

Therapists are often more psychologically minded than clients and can identify the controlling variable(s) in their own chains more quickly. Of course, this generalization needs to be assessed to make sure that therapists' ideas are accurate since they often have blind spots when it comes to understanding their own behavior. Another difference is that team frequently relies on an honor code of sorts, in which the therapists bring up problems for which they need help. Unlike individual therapy, in which both clients and therapists identify problems in need of change, in team, the therapist has to bring up his or her own behavior as a target. These are relatively small differences; there are many commonalities. It turns out that therapists are people too and subject to all the same principles of behavior (effective *and* ineffective) as our clients.

Problems Doing Chains in Teams

Common problems that arise when conducting chains on a team include urges to avoid, defensiveness, rushing to problem solving, and the tendency to treat one another as fragile. These problems are not exclusive to the conduct of chains. Urges to avoid doing chain analysis can occur on the part of every member of a team. The person who engages in a target behavior may feel embarrassed and not want to discuss it, especially in a large group. The team leader, who would likely be conducting the chain, might also be embarrassed about having his or her therapeutic skills on display for others to assess. In addition, the team leader might feel guilty or anxious about confronting a teammate about a target behavior. Other members of a team might wish to avoid chains in order to keep the peace or because they are anxious to get to other topics on the agenda. An obstacle to conducting effective chains on teams involves treating teammates as fragile and not capable of receiving negative feedback. Suggesting that a behavior is in need of a chain analysis often involves confronting a peer or highlighting a behavior that is seen as potentially problematic. There may be a perception that there are greater negative consequences for suggesting a chain be done with a peer as opposed to a client. For all these reasons, it is common for chain analyses to fall to the bottom of the to-do list and for teams to consistently not have time to do them. Therefore, I suggest that teams place chain analyses on the agenda every week so that it is not so easily avoided. Then if any target behavior arises in need of chain analysis, there is place for it within the schedule. The team leader has to take responsibility for providing the rationale for the importance of conducting chain analyses on the team, much like an individual therapist would do in a session.

Another obstacle to the effective use of chains on teams includes defensiveness, which can show up when therapists feels accused of something, singled out, or invalidated. For example, when conducting a chain on lateness, a therapist might say, "Amanda [another team member] was late last week and we didn't do a chain on her!" or a therapist might be quick to offer "valid" reasons for his or her behavior ("I couldn't help it! I was late because my kid was sick!") as justification for not needing to do a chain. Similar to confronting a target behavior, a team member might have to call out defensiveness by ringing an observer bell, for example (see Sayrs, 2019), or return to the rationale of chains in the team by linking them to what happens in therapy.

Finally, as with chains with clients, the team has to watch for rushing into problem solving before the problem has been assessed. The structure of the chain can sometimes be an antidote to this practice since it forces the team to understand different components of the situation before moving on to solutions. However, given that most DBT therapists like to be problem solvers, I have found it very common for teams to stop at each link to offer helpful suggestions. At the risk of sounding like a broken record, I encourage teams to practice chains in the same way as they would in individual sessions; thus, staying mindful about the need to understand the problem before diving in with solutions is critically important.

Tips for Doing Chains in Teams

It's generally advised that one person take the lead and be the assessor. I recommend this method for a couple of reasons. One is that it most mimics what would happen in individual therapy when there is only the therapist and the client and the therapist does the entire chain from start to finish. The second reason is that with many therapists chiming in all at once, there can be a lack of clarity and coherence to the overall chain. Chains can be collaborative endeavors with multiple people asking questions as long as the team leader takes charge. The team leader is responsible for noting when the chain is going in too many directions and for redirecting discussion when necessary. Another option includes therapists doing chains on themselves outside of team (e.g., using the chain analyses worksheets in the skills manual) and then bringing them to team to discuss and ask for input about anything that might be missing. By doing so, time in team is spent on controlling variables and missing information rather than on the attainment of information.

Example of Chain Analysis in Team

Gary has been late to three of the last four team meetings. When he arrives 10 minutes late to this meeting (12:10 P.M.), he is visibly flustered and apologizes as he comes in to the room. Serena, the team leader for the day, turns the conversation to him after they are done discussing an agenda item.

SERENA: Hi, Gary! You being late gives me the perfect opportunity to not avoid difficult tasks. It's hard for me to feel like I'm calling out another team member! Are you willing to let me try a chain here? *(light, easy manner and tone)*

GARY: Ugh, I know. I'm really sorry guys—what can I say, it's an issue for me.

SERENA: What do you mean? You mean you're late for lots of things, not just team meetings?

GARY: Oh yeah, I'm late to almost everything. I know I have major time management issues.

SERENA: Ah, OK, so this team lateness is not unusual for you? It's part of a larger pattern?

GARY: Totally. My wife has been complaining about this flaw for years! *(Laughs.)*

SERENA: OK, well we might not be able to solve your lateness everywhere and it's really important that we're all here on time for team, right? I mean you miss mindfulness when you're a few minutes late and sometimes that's the most important part, at least for me. [orienting to importance of the task and highlighting consequences]

GARY: I know, I know. Mindfulness is really helpful for me.

SERENA: OK, so I'm aware of time and the fact that we have lots of things on our agenda today. I'm wondering if we could do a macro chain on what happened today with your lateness? We could all use the practice of doing these quick and dirty chains. [orienting and providing rationale]

GARY: Sure. I'm game.

SERENA: Great! So how is it that you were late by 10 minutes to team today? [opening question]

GARY: I was just now meeting with my client, Tracy, whom I've discussed in team a lot. She has had a number of crises this past week and it just felt like we didn't have enough time. I'd love to get the team's help with dealing with all the stuff she has going on.

SERENA: OK, we can add you to the agenda for sure. Do you always meet with Tracy before team?

GARY: No, this was a rescheduled meeting. One of the many crises was that her car was in the repair shop, so she couldn't make our typical session time.

SERENA: So you were meeting with her this morning right before team and ran late, but since you don't always meet with her before team *and* you're still often late, it doesn't seem like Tracy having a lot going on is necessarily totally responsible for your lateness. Would you agree? [highlighting that Gary's understanding of the prompting event might not be accurate in terms of controlling variables]

GARY: Yes, I guess that's fair.

SERENA: At what point did you realize you were going to be late for the team? [identifying prompting event]

GARY: *(Looks down, embarrassed.)* Uh, well, it was after Tracy left and I was doing some paperwork.

SERENA: Oh! So what time was that?

GARY: Probably a couple minutes before 12:00. I thought "I should get this session note done now because otherwise I'll forget and it will cause problems for me later." I should have just come to team.

[Team member Anne rings the bell, signaling to all that a judgment was expressed.]

SERENA: Good catch, Anne! Gary, want to state that again without judgment?

GARY: Right. Yes. If I had left just when I saw what time it was, I wouldn't have been late for team.

SERENA: Great. And I think I agree with that! So what happened? It was a couple of minutes before 12:00, you could have made it to team on time if you have just left your office then, but instead you stayed and did your paperwork. So it wasn't just your session running long, though I'm sure that didn't help. Is this the sort of thing that happens with other instances of lateness?

GARY: Yes. I constantly think I have more time than I do to get stuff done. I think I thought I could just whip out a session note and then be a couple of minutes late for team which was no big deal but of course I hit a snag with my computer and then spent a few minutes trying to figure that out, didn't even get the session note done because the computer froze! And here I am.

ANNE: Do you think it's important to be at team on time?

SERENA: Gary not thinking it's that important is a hypothesis, I guess, but just one possibility. What do you think, Gary? Is part of the problem that you don't think it's important to be at team on time? [leader taking control of the chain, avoiding potential judgments by team members]

GARY: No, I don't think so. I think I just have a real deficit when it comes to having realistic expectations for how much I can accomplish in any given time.

SERENA: OK, that's good to know. And you're definitely not the only one with that particular deficit! My husband is the same way! So one last piece: What were the consequences of your team lateness behavior? [assessing consequences]

GARY: *(laughing)* Isn't it obvious? We had to do this chain, didn't we?

SERENA: Well, yes, having to do a chain is a consequence. But I'm trying to get at whether there are any reinforcers to lateness behavior?

GARY: It didn't happen this time but sometimes I do get another task done when I'm late for something.

SERENA: Has that happened with past teams when you've been late, do you think?

GARY: Yeah, I'm sure I've gotten some paperwork accomplished before team on other days that I've been late.

SERENA: And, besides today, maybe the absence of negative consequences has also allowed the behavior to continue?

GARY: Yeah, probably. Though not anymore!

SERENA: Ha! Well it's possible that just knowing you might have another chain done will motivate you to be on time, but I want to try something else too. It's been a few minutes and we have a lot to get to on the agenda. I'm wondering if we can try something for next week just to see how it goes? What if you set an alarm on your phone right now that goes off at 11:55? And no matter what you're doing, you just stop it right there, and come to our group meeting. Can you give that a try?

GARY: Yeah, I can try it. It may actually work! *(laughing)*

SERENA: And if it doesn't, we can do another chain! Why don't you pull out your phone right now to set it?

GARY: OK, sounds good. *(Takes out phone.)*

SERENA: Now let's get to the other items on our agenda . . .

Commentary

This is a short chain with some elements common to other chains discussed in this book as well as some departures. Serena's tone and style is really important in reducing defensiveness and judgments on Gary's part, as well as the rest of team. She provides a rationale for doing a chain in team and uses some self-disclosure (i.e., that doing the chain is good exposure and practice for her) to help increase buy-in. At the same time, Serena assesses fairly quickly the main components of the chain. Although the problem of lateness for Gary more broadly is not addressed in this chain, the calling attention to the behavior and identifying a solution likely increases his awareness, as well as that of other team members. Doing the chain in team, as opposed to talking with Gary individually outside of the team, also functions to make lateness behavior a team problem, rather than an individual clinician's problem. Many of these elements are true when discussing the use of chains in skills training groups as well.

Use of Chain Analysis in Skills Training

Aside from any specific week in which the skill of chain analysis is taught, chains are used sparingly in skills training. The primary reason for this is that time spent on chains, even when they are addressing therapy-interfering behavior, is often time taken away from skills training. The skills trainer has to be mindful of the target hierarchy for skills training and how it differs from the target hierarchy in individual therapy. In skills training, the target hierarchy is (1) eliminate therapy-destroying behavior, (2) increase skills acquisition, and (3) decrease therapy-interfering behaviors (Linehan, 1993, 2015). The goal is to have few, if any, therapy-destroying behaviors, which means that the vast majority of skills training is spent on skills teaching, review, and practice. Most of the time, therapy-interfering behavior, if addressed at all in group, is highlighted without going into depth with a chain analysis (e.g., a skills group later might say, "You're late again! Please try to get here on time next week, OK?").

There are times, however, when therapy-interfering behavior rises to the point where addressing it could be a teaching opportunity. It can effectively weave together assessment and problem solving in a manner that is beneficial to multiple members of the group. The person who is engaging in the behavior has the opportunity to "tell his or her story" and understand the factors that contribute to the occurrence of the behavior, and the other group members have the opportunity to learn something about the process of conducting chains.

For example, much like in team meetings, as discussed above, a frequent problem in skills training is lateness. If skills trainers don't attend to lateness, it quickly can become a pattern of behavior that is highly disruptive. Lateness behavior also frequently communicates to others that lateness is OK and the norm of being on time is no longer emphasized or supported. A skills trainer tells a client's individual therapist about the lateness, so it gets addressed in individual therapy. The individual therapist might be working hard on reducing lateness behavior but that is not necessarily known to anyone else in the group and, in the meantime, the lateness continues. Thus, doing a macro chain on the lateness in group could strengthen what is happening in individual therapy and also communicate to everyone else in group that this is an important issue for the group as a whole. Other behaviors that might provide the context for a macro chain in group include not doing one's homework or not bringing one's materials to group (both conceptualized as "missing effective behaviors") or leaving the room repeatedly during group. Importantly, when doing a chain in the context of skills group, the leader has to keep it short, succinct, and focused on the principle of returning to skills training as quickly as possible. As much as possible, the leader also wants to involve the other group members in some way so that they aren't just sitting back. This runs the risk of their seeing the discussion as irrelevant to them. If a leader does not have confidence that he or she could achieve a brief chain given the complexity of the target behavior, then he or she should not do the chain in group; instead she should bring up the behavior at consultation team and discuss options for how to address it. Furthermore, if the target behavior involves a potential or real conflict between group members, a chain on that behavior in group should be avoided and redirected toward individual therapy.

Example of Chain Analysis in a Skills Training Group

Lisa is a skills group leader who has noticed a pattern of lateness in her group. Over the past few weeks, there has been a tendency for only two or three members to be present at the start of group, with the other members slowly trickling in. This pattern makes the beginning of group feel disjointed, with Lisa often having to repeat herself several times, and Dan, the co-leader, having to leave the room several times to try to track down missing members. These behaviors are interfering with teaching. Thus, Lisa planfully decides that she will do a chain of a late member in group in order to both address the problem for that particular member and to signal to the other members in the group that being on time is important and that there is a potential consequence for arriving late. She knows in advance that she doesn't want to spend more than 5 minutes total on it.

The group start time is 7:00 P.M. and, like in past groups, only two members are present at the start. Two others arrive at 7:05, one at 7:15, and then Tina arrives at 7:30. At the time that Tina arrives, Lisa is reviewing the homework of Rob, another member. She glances up at Tina, warmly says, "Hi Tina, so glad you made it," finishes up the homework review with Rob, and then says to Tina:

LISA: Tina, we're reviewing everyone's homework and I want to get to yours in a second. However, I wanted to spend a few minutes trying to figure out what happened with you being late today! Group, have you noticed that we're having a problem with lateness? (*Group members nod.*) So I'm thinking we can use wonderful Tina here for a quick chain analysis to see what's getting in the way of being here on time. And I promise to keep it short and sweet, OK?

TINA: (*Looks embarrassed, eyes down, blushing.*) Do we have to?

LISA: We don't have to—let's just see how it goes, OK? [not spending time on avoidance/reasons for not wanting to] So what happened? How is it that you're 30 minutes late today?

TINA: I just really didn't want to come. I was in bed and my mother kept telling me I had to get up and come and I just felt like I couldn't do it. Then she called my therapist who helped me come.

LISA: Oh, this is so wonderful! I'm so glad that you came even though you didn't want to. Does this ever happen to other people—having a really hard time getting yourself to come to group? [involving other members]

OTHERS: Yes, all the time.

LISA: So this is a common problem and I'm guessing it has come up for you at other times, Tina, not just tonight, right?

TINA: Yeah.

LISA: So it's worth trying to figure out what happened so we can get it to go differently next time and be on time to group. [orienting to chain and also to target behavior] At what point did you know you were going to be late tonight? [anchoring in time, looking for prompting event]

TINA: When it was 6:30 and I hadn't left the house yet.

LISA: OK, and what was happening then? What were you doing and thinking?

TINA: I was lying in bed, watching videos on my laptop.

LISA: And thinking?

TINA: "I should get up and go to group."

LISA: What were you feeling?

TINA: Depressed and kinda hopeless.

LISA: OK, so sadness maybe?

TINA: Yeah, pretty sad.

LISA: The good news is that we're going to be talking about observing and describing emotions today, so we're getting a head start. In fact, we may return to this example later if it would be helpful. [linking to skills training] So you were in bed, not getting up, though you were having thoughts to do so. Sounds like your thoughts and your emotions and urges were fighting.

TINA: Yeah, they were.

LISA: So then what happened?

TINA: My mom started to call to me, "Tina, time to go to group," and that sort of just made me angry. I yelled at her that she should leave me alone and that I'm in charge of my own life. Then she busted into the room and held out her phone and my therapist was on it.

LISA: OK, and then what happened? [choosing not to go into more detail about any of those links given time constraints]

TINA: I talked to my therapist and she told me to use opposite action to get out of bed and drive here. She made me stay on the phone with her until I got in the car.

LISA: Oh, I love that! What were you thinking and feeling as you were talking to your therapist?

TINA: Honestly, a little annoyed, but I kinda just went through the motions. She told me that when I'm using opposite action, I have to try not to think too much.

LISA: I get that. And for the rest of you, if you don't know it yet, never fear, we'll be getting to opposite action in just a couple of weeks. Tina is demonstrating a great use of it—basically acting opposite to the urges to stay in bed by getting up and out of the house. [involving other members, linking to skills teaching] So then you got here at 7:30. I'm wondering if you can name any of the consequences for being late?

TINA: Having to do this chain in front of everyone!

LISA: Well that's true—is that a positive or negative experience for you? [not assuming]

TINA: Very negative.

LISA: OK, so we'll remember that. [not spending time on this link for now—just observing it] Any other consequences you can think of?

TINA: No.

LISA: What about other people? Can you think of other consequences of being late? [involving the group—also making it a bit more generic in order to assess general consequences for lateness]

OTHER MEMBER: I hate feeling all scattered when I get here later and feeling like I missed stuff.

ANOTHER MEMBER: You don't get to hear how others' homework went.

LISA: Really great, you guys. The others I can think of are missing mindfulness and also our poor co-leader Dan has to leave group to track everyone down. Oh and also we all worry when you aren't here! [naming consequences that might not be apparent to all the group members] (Turns toward Tina.) So, I'm so glad that you talked to your therapist and practiced opposite action to get here. That's really excellent and I'm glad you're here now for the rest of group. One last thing—what can you do differently next week when you're feeling similar urges to avoid before group?

TINA: I could practice opposite action earlier, I guess.

LISA: (dramatic) Yes!! That's the best idea I've heard. Anyone else have suggestions? [involving others]

DAN [co-leader]: What about doing something pleasant right before group? Like what if you stopped to get a nice tea somewhere on your way to group?

TINA: Oh yeah, that's a good idea. Like my reward for getting up and going?

DAN: Right.

TINA: I can do that.

LISA: Excellent. So write that down in your notebook. We'll all be so excited to see you at 6:55 P.M. next week. And everyone else too! Now, moving on . . . (*Goes to next person for homework review.*)

Commentary

This was an illustration of a typical short chain that might occur in skills training to address therapy-interfering behavior. There were numerous instances when the therapist might have stopped to get more information, but instead she kept her eye on having this be a brief macro chain that gets some of the major components of the chain so that a solution or two could be generated. In many instances, these group macro chains end up highlighting lots of areas in which skills training can be incorporated. Thus, the therapist looks for opportunities to link to the skills being taught in the current group or upcoming groups. One thing that may be different in chains that occur in the group format is that the therapist has to be sensitive to possible embarrassment and shame that occurs when a problem is highlighted in a public setting. Therefore, another strategy that a therapist can use is to normalize as much as possible and relate the problem being discussed to everyone else in group. Maintaining an easy manner is important, as is reinforcement of adaptive behaviors as much as possible.

Use of Chain Analysis in Phone Coaching

Similar to skills training, the use of chains during a phone-coaching call is minimal. To review, the target hierarchy in phone calls is to reduce suicide crises, increase skills generalization, and decrease therapy relationship conflict. Therefore, a therapist doesn't go into a phone call with a client thinking that he or she will be doing a fine-grained chain analysis. What is unique about the available opportunities in phone calls is that ideally a client is calling in the middle of the chain, that is, before he or she has engaged in ineffective behaviors. Therefore, the therapist is helping to steer the chain in a more effective direction. Assessment that occurs in a phone call is going to be brief and focused, with a eye toward changing the path of the immediate future.

That said, it is often helpful for therapists to keep the structure of the chain in mind. With clients who are familiar with the process of chains, the language can be incorporated into the call. For example, a therapist can ask, "What was the prompting event for this spike in urges to harm yourself?" or "Any particular vulnerability factors for you today?" This kind of question often functions to get important information quickly. The therapist can also highlight important (negative) consequences for the target behavior that have been learned from prior chains (e.g., "I know your urges to avoid going to school are really high right now and we both know from recent experiences that if you don't go, you'll end up feeling a lot more depressed later with more work piled up"). While the assessment is notably briefer during phone-coaching calls, the emphasis on the sequence of events remains the same.

Importantly, phone-coaching calls are often referred to in the next individual session. Thus, the events that are occuring in the person's life leading to the phone call would likely be addressed in a more formal chain in the subsequent therapy session. The phone call is giving the therapist some insight into important links at the time they are happening, which can aid him or her later in a more comprehensive assessment. For example, the client during a session might report having difficulty remembering what he was thinking during his highly dysregulated state, but the therapist might remember certain thoughts he was expressing at the time of the call and use that information to flesh out the chain.

Example of Chain Analysis in a Phone-Coaching Call

Although this example is a fairly typical phone-coaching session, I highlight ways in which a chain analysis is conducted. Greg, a 17-year-old client with recurrent self-harm behavior in the form of cutting with razors, texts his therapist, Diana, at 9:00 P.M. He states that he is "feeling miserable" and "doesn't know what to do." Diana responds that it sounds like he could use some phone coaching and asks him to call her. He calls her about 30 minutes later.

DIANA: Hi, Greg, I'm glad you called! What's happening?

GREG: I'm feeling really agitated and miserable.

DIANA: Where are you and what are you are doing?

GREG: I'm in my room. I was trying to listen to music but it feels like nothing is working.

DIANA: Are you having urges to harm yourself? [assessing target behavior]

GREG: Yeah, they're pretty strong.

DIANA: Have you harmed yourself?

GREG: No, not yet.

DIANA: OK, that's great. Though I don't like the sound of "not yet." We're going to get this to go differently so that the answer is a definitive "No, and I'm not going to," OK?

GREG: OK.

DIANA: What are your urges right now on a 0 to 5 scale?

GREG: 5.

DIANA: And do you have anything to cut yourself with?

GREG: There's a razor in the bathroom I'm sure, but there's nothing in my room.

DIANA: Great. OK, so what set these urges off? What's your best guess as to the prompting event? [using chain terms to identify prompting event for urges]

GREG: Sarah [girlfriend] and I got in a fight.

DIANA: When did that happen?

GREG: A couple hours ago. I asked her to come over and she said no because she had a test to study for and somehow this turned into her accusing me of only wanting to spend time with her for sex.

DIANA: [purposely not assessing some of these more specific links] Sounds like a difficult conversation! I'm sure we'll talk more about that on Wednesday [the next scheduled session], but now I'm curious about what emotions you were experiencing during the fight and then after?

GREG: I was angry during the fight and we said some nasty stuff to each other. But then I felt ashamed and now I'm thinking she's going to break up with me and I f—ked up another relationship.

DIANA: OK, good labeling of those painful emotions. So anger and shame sound pretty intense. When did the urge to harm yourself first show up?

GREG: Pretty soon after I got off the phone.

DIANA: Which was how long ago?

GREG: About an hour.

DIANA: And what have you been doing to manage your urges so far? [assessing functional links in the chain, given that he hasn't self-harmed]

GREG: I texted you. Put on some music. But I'm just lying in bed now feeling terrible.

DIANA: Does that mean replaying the argument in your head and thinking about her ending the relationship?

GREG: Yeah, and what that means for me—like how I'm going to be alone forever and all that. And how worthless I am.

DIANA: OK, so then the thoughts spiral. I'm so glad you called me. Let me summarize what I think you're saying and see if I have all the facts right so that we can move into what you need to do next, OK?

GREG: OK.

DIANA: A couple hours ago you were talking to Sarah, asked her to come over, and she said no. This turned into an argument about your relationship during which she accused you of only wanting her for sex. This led to you feeling angry and ashamed and having thoughts that she might end the relationship. You then tried a few skillful things like calling me and listening to music, but your urges to self-harm are still pretty strong and now we need to figure out something else to do that will help you feel better or at least tolerate the situation without self-harming. Do you think I have that right?

GREG: Yeah, you got it.

Commentary

This assessment portion of the phone call likely took about 5 minutes to complete and now Diana and Greg turn to solutions, that is, skills that Greg can use in the moment to change the chain of events toward effective behaviors. The therapist used chain analysis language when assessing and also kept clear the sequence of events as she assessed. She also helpfully summarized the sequence of events for the client and made sure she understood it correctly before moving on to offer specific help. This summary is often necessary to ensure that the client and the therapist are on the same page so that the offered solutions are the ones that are most likely to work. If the therapist doesn't understand the situation sufficiently, there is greater risk that he or she will offer solutions that won't help the problem. Notice that in this example, Diana did not spend time assessing vulnerability factors or consequences in this chain. Vulnerability information may be useful in understanding why the urges to self-harm showed up in this particular context, and therefore might be useful for more long-term solutions; however, it is unlikely to affect the instructions for the next few minutes. Consequences were not assessed because Greg had not engaged in the target behavior and was, in fact, calling before consequences could occur.

This chapter focused on the ways in which chain analyses are incorporated into the other modes of DBT. I discussed strategies for how to keep them short and focused while still maintaining the structural integrity. These "macro chains" are incredibly useful in multiple situations in which more in-depth chains are not possible or preferred. Team consultation meetings provide good opportunities to practice these macro chains in order to learn how to skillfully get to the heart of the matter quickly. These skills can then be artfully applied in skills training groups and phone coaching calls when time is of the essence.

In this book, I have reviewed the basics of chain analysis, how to use the assessment method across a wide variety of target behaviors, situations, and settings, and how to incorporate other important DBT strategies. It is my hope that this book greatly expands the literature on clinical applications of DBT and provides helpful instruction for how to apply chain analysis with fidelity. By doing so, the client's target behaviors will be more fully understood, which will lead to more effective solution generation and better outcomes.

References

Heard, H. L., & Swales, M. A. (2015). *Changing behavior in DBT: Problem solving in action.* New York: Guilford Press.

Koerner, K. (2011). *Doing dialectical behavior therapy: A practical guide.* New York: Guilford Press.

Linehan, M. M. (1993). *Cognitive-behavioral treatment of borderline personality disorder.* New York: Guilford Press.

Linehan, M. M. (1997). Validation and psychotherapy. In A. Bohart & L. Greenberg (Eds.), *Empathy reconsidered: New directions in psychotherapy* (pp. 353–392). Washington, DC: American Psychological Association.

Linehan, M. M. (2015). *DBT skills training manual* (2nd ed.). New York: Guilford Press.

Linehan, M. M., & Wilks, C. R. (2015). The course and evolution of dialectical behavior therapy. *American Journal of Psychotherapy, 69,* 97–110.

Lynch, T. R., Chapman, A. L., Rosenthal, M. Z., Kuo, J. R., & Linehan, M. M. (2006). Mechanisms of change in dialectical behavior therapy: Theoretical and empirical observations. *Journal of Clinical Psychology, 62*(4), 459–480.

Rizvi, S. L., & Roman, K. M. (2019). Generalization modalities: Taking the treatment out of the consulting room—using telephone, text, and email. In M. A. Swales (Ed.), *The Oxford handbook of dialectical behaviour therapy* (pp. 201–216). Oxford, UK: Oxford University Press.

Rizvi, S. L., & Sayrs, J. H. (2018). Assessment-driven case formulation and treatment planning in dialectical behavior therapy: Using principles to guide effective treatment. *Cognitive and Behavioral Practice.* Retrieved from *www.sciencedirect.com/science/article/pii/S1077722917300718.* [Epub ahead of print]

Sayrs, J. H. R. (2019). Running an effective DBT consultation team: Principles and challenges. In M. A. Swales (Ed.), *The Oxford handbook of dialectical behaviour therapy* (pp. 147–166). Oxford, UK: Oxford University Press.

Swenson, C. R. (2016). *DBT principles in action: Acceptance, change, and dialectics.* New York: Guilford Press.

Williams, H. L., Conway, M. A., & Cohen, G. (2008). Autobiographical memory. In G. Cohen & M. Conway (Eds.), *Memory in the real world* (3rd ed., pp. 21–90). New York: Psychology Press.

Index

Note. *f* or *t* following a page number indicates a figure or a table.